Is It Sensory or Is It Behavior?

Behavior Problem Identification, Assessment, and Intervention

Carolyn Murray-Slutsky,
MS, OTR

Betty A. Paris, PT, M.Ed.

H HAMMILL INSTITUTE ON DISABILITIES
8700 SHOAL CREEK BOULEVARD
AUSTIN, TEXAS 78757-6897
512/451-3521   FAX 512/451-3728

HAMMILL INSTITUTE ON DISABILITIES
8700 SHOAL CREEK BOULEVARD
AUSTIN, TEXAS 78757-6897
512/451-3521   FAX 512/451-3728

The Library of Congress has cataloged the original paperback edition as follows:

Murray-Slutsky, Carolyn, 1953—
   Is it sensory or is it behavior? : behavior problem identification, assessment, and intervention / Carolyn Murray-Slutsky, Petty Paris.
         p. cm.
   Includes bibliographical references.
      ISBN 0-7616-421-0 (pbk)
   1. Behavior disorders in children—Etiology. 2. Behavior disorders in children—Diagnosis. 3. Behavior disorders in children—Treatment. 4. Sensory integration dysfunction in children. 5. Problem children—Behavior modification. 6. Behavior therapy for children. 7. Conditioned response.
      [DNLM: 1. Child Behavior Disorders—etiology. 2. Child Behavior Disorders—therapy. 3. Sensory Thresholds—physiology. WS 350.6 M984i 2005] I. Paris, Betty A., 1952- II. Title.
RJ506.B44M87 2005
618.92'89—dc22

2005011153

Current Hammill Institute on Disabilities ISBN-13: 978-160251006-7
Current Hammill Institute on Disabilities ISBN-10: 160251006-7

Previously published by PsychCorp, a division of Harcourt Assessment, Inc., under ISBN 0761644210.

Printed in the United States of America

3 4 5 6   11 10 09 08

About the Authors

Carolyn Murray-Slutsky, MS, OTR, is director and founder of Rehabilitation for Children, a pediatric private practice. She co-founded M P Rehabilitative Services, a pediatric private practice that specialized in outpatient, home, and school-based therapy in Florida, which was acquired by a national corporation in 2001. Carolyn received her undergraduate degree in special education from Ohio University and her master's degree in occupational therapy from Boston University.

Carolyn is certified in sensory integration (SI) and neurodevelopmental treatment (NDT) for pediatrics, infants, and adults. Her work experience includes more than twenty years working in direct patient care and in consultative, educational, and administrative positions. She is also an adjunct professor teaching occupational and physical therapy students.

She received the Manager of the Year award while serving as director of rehabilitation for an acute-care facility. In 1999 she was honored with the Award of Excellence by the Florida Occupational Therapy Association for her long-standing and significant contributions to the occupational therapy profession.

Betty A. Paris, PT, M.Ed., attained her bachelor of science degree in physical therapy from Florida International University and her master's in education from the University of Phoenix.

Betty holds certificates in SI and NDT in pediatrics and babies. She has used her dual certificates to develop a unique blend of NDT and SI treatments offered to children and young adults in a variety of settings and has shared this with therapists, parents, and other professionals through educational seminars.

Her professional experience includes a wide range of venues including hospitals, community-based services, and private practice. Betty has used her expertise, dual certifications in NDT and SI, and her M.Ed. as an adjunct professor to offer online programs to occupational and physical therapy students.

Paris and Murray-Slutsky, together with Herman Slutsky, have formed STAR Services, a company dedicated to providing high-quality educational and consultative services. Paris and Murray-Slutsky lecture throughout the United States and internationally. Their presentations offer state-of-the-art treatment methods in topics related to SI, NDT, functional therapy, behavior, and splinting techniques designed to give participants the skills and techniques needed to improve the functional performance of children with sensory and neurological problems. They are authors of the Therapy Skill Builders textbook *Exploring the Spectrum of Autism and Pervasive Developmental Disorders: Intervention Strategies,* which provides practical holistic intervention strategies.

Contributor

Mary M. Murray, Ed.D.
Assistant Professor
Specialized Education Services
Early Childhood Special Education
University of North Carolina at Greensboro
mmmurray@buckeye-express.com

Equipment Contributors

Southpaw Enterprises®. Provides sensory, motor, and educational products for therapeutic professionals, teachers, and parents, and is dedicated to the advancement of sensory integration.

P.O. Box 1047
Dayton, Ohio 45401-1047
1-800-228-1698
www.southpawenterprises.com

Abilitations. Part of Sportime International, a dynamic, innovative catalog company that provides movement activity products, equipment, and sensory products designed specifically for the changing needs of children. Their catalogues include *SpaceKraft*, *Integrations,* and *Sportime.*

P.O. Box 620856
Atlanta, Georgia 30362
1-800-850-8602
www.abilitations.com

Table of Contents

List of Figures

List of Tables

Acknowledgments

We would like to express our gratitude to all the people who have shared their expertise and helped to make this book possible. To Southpaw Enterprises®, for their support and promotion of sensory integration, thank you for your dedication to our profession.

Thanks also go to Laura Clahane, an outstanding teacher in the autism cluster at Pembroke Pines Charter Elementary School, whose positive behavioral support of her children is inspirational; Marta Maldonado; and Mary Martin who, together with Ms. Clahane, make a wonderful, caring team.

To Abilitations, thank you for your support of our educational endeavors.

We extend our gratitude to the parents of the children we treat. Your energy and dedication to helping your children have been an inspiration and compelling force behind our effort to help you. By entrusting us with the care of your children, sharing your trials and tribulations, as well as your successes, you have contributed to our growth as professionals and individuals.

To the children we treat, we are emboldened by your trust and the insights you have shared with us. Thank you for allowing us to share in your experiences and your triumphs.

To the practitioners and professionals in our field, we thank all the therapists who have worked for and with us over the years and all the participants of our workshops. You have fueled our determination to tease out viable solutions to the complexities of behavior that we all face in the children we treat. Your questions have helped us identify the problems facing us, forced us to research different techniques and theories, and helped crystallize our own beliefs in developing our treatment strategies. Your feedback on the effectiveness of our philosophies and techniques, and your encouragement to put those theories and beliefs into print, have been a driving force behind this book.

Thank you to all the teachers, educational specialists, behavioralists, and physicians who saw a difference in our interventions and the objective improvements in the children, and who encouraged us to share our knowledge with others.

Thanks to everyone at Myrland Stables in Davie, Florida, for their continual help, their love of horses, their endless advice and support, and their drive to be better than they are. Special thanks to Pam Southerton, Sherry Morris, Brook Wood, Pat Lezaca, Joan Mulligan, Richard Weissman, Jo Ann Bennett, Brenda Tsgaris, Lee Schoenberg, Ann Margaret Mastropaolo, and Steven and Linda Duchac.

To our own families, thank you for your unconditional love and understanding, and for tolerating the unending hours of work in the search for knowledge and answers. Thanks especially to Herman, for your admiration and belief in us—your help and support has enabled us to complete this and so many other projects. Thanks to Steve, for your unending support and strength; to David, Stephanie, and Jerry for your encouragement and understanding; and to Mom and Dad for your constant support and encouragement. Without your sacrifices, support, assistance, and love, this book would not have been possible.

Preface

We began our clinical practice in pediatrics over twenty years ago, addressing the needs of the children we saw using primarily motor control treatment strategies. The *Sensory Integration and Praxis Test* was just being developed, as were training and certification programs in sensory integration. As we strived to understand the concepts being proposed and developed by A. J. Ayres, so we struggled to integrate the new knowledge with our use and understanding of motor control and neurodevelopmental treatment (NDT) techniques. We were convinced that the holistic approach provided by the use of the two techniques was an important breakthrough in clinical practice and wanted to share our experiences and knowledge with other therapists.

As we began lecturing to therapists on integrating NDT and sensory integration techniques in the early 1990s through the American Occupational Therapy Association, we were bombarded by questions regarding children's behaviors, the possible underlying causes of those behaviors, and what could be done to address them. We continue to be asked those same questions today. As we travel the world over, we find that behavior is one of the most complex and pertinent issues on the minds of therapists today.

We disagreed with those who believed that sensory behaviors could be addressed only from a sensory perspective. Brad, a seven-year-old boy who was referred to us due to sensory processing concerns, strangled children when he became overstimulated by people and things in his environment. His parents believed that he could not be held accountable because his behavior stemmed from sensory processing difficulties. The only remediation was to treat the underlying sensory processing problem and hope the strangling behavior stopped.

We witnessed sensory diets being prescribed that provided the child with sensory stimulation, not the sensory integration so sorely needed. Some sensory diets also allowed the child to avoid the demands placed upon him or her, work at school, or compliance at home. We believe wholeheartedly in sensory diets, but posed the question as to how and when they are to be used. We worked to determine where sensory diets fit into treatment regimens, and how not to allow them to serve for task avoidance.

We encountered behaviorists who believed that a behavioral approach was the only way to address behaviors, whether or not they were sensory. But we saw that when a sensory-based behavior was extinguished using solely behavioral techniques, a new and often more alarming behavior emerged.

In our first book, *Exploring the Spectrum of Autism and Pervasive Developmental Disorders: Intervention Strategies* (Murry-Slutsky and Paris 2000), we began to look at behaviors as they are expressed and related to the autism spectrum disorders. We were inundated with questions regarding children who did not fall into the autism spectrum and were driven by the need to look at and write about how to deal with the behaviors of children with other conditions.

As so often happens in life, fate took a twist that would affect how we looked at, interpreted, and dealt with sensory behaviors in children. Carolyn befriended a horse named

Rusty. His mannerisms and behaviors would ultimately lead Carolyn and me to look at behaviors from a fresh, new perspective. Over the next two years, we looked at behaviors in many different ways as we worked to unravel the myriad of challenging behaviors exhibited by Rusty. Carolyn's story, and our lesson follows.

Rusty, a Lesson in Sensory Behavior

Is it sensory or is it behavior? That was the question I posed to Steven Duchac, our horse trainer in Ocala, Florida. He answered, "Rusty is all sensory, but his sensory problems come out as behavior problems." I was more amazed that Steven understood my question than by the answer. After all, it is a question that we, as pediatric therapists, are frequently called upon to answer. Steven's answer struck a cord.

I fell in love with Rusty because of his problems; I was drawn to him because I understood him and instinctively knew what he needed. Rusty's behaviors mirrored many of those seen in children with sensory integrative disorders. Working with him strengthened my knowledge of sensory integration and my belief that behaviors, whether sensory or otherwise, can and must be dealt with.

I first met Rusty in April 2001. My husband, Herman, and I had just returned from a horseback-riding trip in Ireland. The trip was so exhilarating that we wanted to continue riding when we returned. At Myrland Stables in Davie, Florida, we learned that we could lease horses on a monthly basis. I was matched up with Rusty, who was new to the stable. They had tried using him for lessons, but felt he would do better with only one rider. He did not adjust well to change, and having different riders was difficult for him.

I vividly remember meeting Rusty for the first time. I went to his stall and called his name. There he stood in the back corner of the stall shaking in fright. I almost cried. I had never seen such a huge animal so scared. What could have happened to him to make him this frightened? I started working with him slowly, and as the weeks and months went by he relaxed and even started to poke his head out the stall door to find out what was going on outside in the world. I knew I had made a breakthrough the day he whinnied to me.

Rusty needed more than just to get to know me. As I got to know Rusty I realized he had some predictable patterns in common with many of the children I treat for sensory integrative dysfunction. Rusty had such high anxiety levels that almost anything would set him off. This was very dangerous to him and those around him. When frightened or spooked, he would jump, turn 180 degrees, and run. Just as the parents of children with sensory integrative disorders do, I learned to anticipate what would set him off and became very adept at handling him. Many people at the stable mislabeled him as a "hyper" horse because of his high anxiety and difficult behaviors. My knowledge of sensory integration led me to believe differently. Instead, he was difficult to get moving in the riding ring. Rusty had low tone and arousal levels. He was all-or-none. It would take me hours to get him to move, and when I finally got him moving, I couldn't get him to stop or slow down. Just as with a child with a modulation disorder, there was no middle ground. Once he started to trot, he would move right into a fast gallop. There was no such thing as a slow canter—he only knew a gallop. I soon realized that he had problems regulating his arousal level; he was either on, or he was off.

Rusty was also clumsy and awkward. He frequently tripped for no reason. It was as if he didn't know he had feet. He moved them automatically but he would trip when there was nothing there to trip on. I felt that he did better after he had been exercised and ridden for a while. His muscle tone increased and his responsiveness was definitely better. He seemed to pick up his feet better and, overall, seemed better coordinated. I found that if I could exercise him before riding, his arousal level and coordination improved and I could ride him safely. The heavy work and exercise definitely helped. I also found that Rusty did much better when I was in the saddle. The extra weight on his back seemed to calm him down and help him organize himself. I was his very own weighted vest!

We heard rumors that before he came to our stable, he had gotten tangled in barbed wire and cut his legs and hoof. That might explain some of his unusual reactions. He has a real fear of gates. He panics and becomes unmanageable in anticipation of passing through a gate. He can't think or listen when he gets into this state. Because of this, the stable help are afraid of him and refuse to put him out in the pasture. All the other horses get turned out every day. Rusty's behavior deprives him of the opportunity to get the exercise he so dearly needs. People are afraid of him and avoid him.

We went through a phase with Rusty where his ornery personality came out and his behavior worsened. He started nipping and biting everyone. He became headstrong and would try to do what he wanted to do when he wanted to do it. Again, his behaviors were interfering with his ability to interact with others and with our efforts to take care of him. The behaviors had to be addressed. We worked through this, but only with a lot of effort.

When summer came he was more sluggish than usual. I noticed that he had trouble breathing and his nostrils would flare after only a slight workout. Eventually it was pointed out to me that he was a *non-sweater*. In the heat, his system shuts down and he does not sweat. Breathing heavily was his only way to attempt to cool his body down. I don't know why I was surprised. I knew he had regulatory problems, just as children with fluctuating arousal levels and self-regulation difficulties often have internal systemic problems that are causing the behavior problems.

The treatment for being a non-sweater is to supplement his grain or feed with a special drink. This sounds easy. But I learned that Rusty wouldn't eat anything that tasted or smelled different. Rusty was demonstrating oral and gustatory (smell) defensive behaviors! The drink was impossible to get down him. He would turn his lips up, show his teeth and make a terrible face. He would stop eating for days. We found the supplement in powdered form and camouflaged it in his grain.

A long-haired horse in South Florida who doesn't sweat is a problem. I decided to shave Rusty in an attempt to help him regulate his body temperature. By this time, I was convinced that Rusty was underresponsive to most sensory input. He had a poor body scheme and panicked when he couldn't predict what was going to happen. He loved being brushed hard and responded well to being handled firmly. People at the stable thought that he would not tolerate the shaver, but I was sure I wouldn't have any problem with the vibration of the shaver. Rusty stood quietly during the four hours it took to shave him. He relaxed the most when the shaver was on his face and nuzzled me for more when I moved to other parts of his body. To everyone's amazement Rusty eventually fell asleep as a result of the vibration.

Joan and Brook, the owners of Myrland stables, brought Steven and Linda Duchac to town, to teach classes in horse training. They used the John Lyons method of horse training, a gentle persuasion technique that had become famous through the popular novel *The Horse Whisperer*. This technique focuses on understanding the horse and getting the horse to want to comply, rather than forcing him to do what you want. Herman and Rusty enrolled in the first three-day clinic.

Rusty quickly earned his reputation for behaving badly. He broke loose and had a panic attack with all the new people at the stable. Steven quickly caught him and taught us how to deal with Rusty's behaviors. We were amazed, but the strategies were familiar. They addressed the horse's sensory systems. Heavy work (proprioceptive and vestibular input) was a key component. I listened and absorbed as much information as I could. After the class we practiced everything we learned.

Six months later they offered the class again. This time I enrolled with Rusty. Steven couldn't believe it was the same horse. Rusty was the model horse for the basics, but we needed to learn more. I absorbed everything I could. I knew it worked. It was sensory integration at its best. I couldn't thank Steven or Rusty enough for what they taught me. They taught me to be a beginner again, to feel the anxiety of not being sure what to do when faced with a difficult behavior. I learned to look at problems through new eyes. Behaviors were broken down into small manageable steps. Sensory principles were integrated into horse training to explain the needs and behaviors of horses. My sensory integrative theory enhanced the horse training, and the horse training expanded my ability to understand the children I treat.

Herman and I had told ourselves we would never buy Rusty. We knew his weaknesses. Who would ever buy a horse like this? Nonetheless, how can you walk away from an animal that has enriched your lives and taught you so much? In April 2003 we became the proud owners of Rusty.

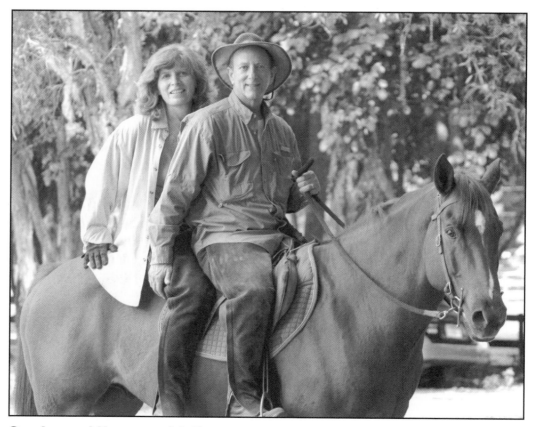

Carolyn and Herman with Rusty.

Our Philosophy on Behavior

The horse-training experiences reinforced our belief that sensory and behavioral issues are intermingled and often cannot be separated. Challenging behaviors, in a horse or child, should seldom be excused, even if sensory issues cause them. Heavy work, as a consequence for negative sensory behaviors, addresses both the behaviors and the underlying sensory issue. As pediatric therapists we believe that behaviors that are sensory in origin are still behaviors and must be dealt with. To excuse unacceptable or socially inappropriate behaviors because they are sensory in nature is a mistake and does the child a disservice. Behaviors interfere with the child's acceptance and interactions within his or her environment and serve only to deprive the child of important learning opportunities and pleasurable life experiences.

In looking at the issues surrounding children and their behavior, we have come to believe that behaviors are very complex and result from multiple causes. They cannot be successfully addressed in a linear fashion, adopting a single strategy to meet the needs served by the behavior. Children make the most rapid increases when behavior and sensory issues are considered together. In Brad's case (the child who strangled children when he became overstimulated by things in his environment), addressing the underlying sensory issues resulting in his overstimulation should decrease his behavior of strangling other children. However, it may take a long time for therapy to take effect and alter this high priority behavior. In the meantime, Brad has learned that strangling others is an effective behavior to alter his environment, deal with his overarousal, and get immediate attention from others—all positive reinforcers to keep the behavior active. This is a learned behavior to cope with his sensory issues.

Brad needs to be taught that strangling is unacceptable and will not be tolerated. Any movement toward strangling a child must result in a consequence. That consequence needs to be sensory and geared toward helping him regain control and organization. Proprioceptive or heavy work activities, such as arm push-ups or table push-ups, frequently are calming and organizing and serve as an effective consequence and self-regulation strategy. The intensity of the exercise must be sufficient to affect his nervous system. This strategy, if implemented after the behavior is exhibited, is reactive. If the workload is difficult enough, it will be effective in addressing both the sensory and learned components of the behavior *after* it has occurred.

Our goal, however, must be to be proactive and prevent the strangling from occurring in the first place. Sensory diets are a proactive approach involving strategically placed activities that will calm Brad's nervous system throughout the day to prevent him from reaching the point of needing to strangle another child. Environmental modifications are another tactic that must be used in a proactive program aimed at prevention. Recognizing and rewarding on-task, appropriate behavior and self-initiated attempts at self-regulation to avoid overarousal and undesirable behavior must also be part of a multipronged prevention program. This type of nonlinear approach to behavior is what we profess. Our goal is to aid families, teachers, and others in dealing with the complexities that behaviors pose.

Is It Sensory or Is It Behavior? 1

Is It Behavior?

Behavioral concerns arise when children's behaviors are bothersome, interfere with their ability to learn or function, or are harmful. These behaviors may include acting without thinking; fidgeting; inattention; distractibility; lack of cooperation; whining, crying, or throwing a tantrum; or aggressive acts, such as pushing, striking out, biting, or hitting. When we ask ourselves, *Is it behavioral?* one of the questions we are asking is, *Is it willful?* Willful implies that the child knows what he or she did, that the child made a conscious decision to act that way (did it on purpose), or that the behavior is within the child's control. Believing a behavior is willful often conjures up emotions and feelings of anger in the person analyzing the behavior because it implies that the child meant to do it.

Behaviors are often *learned* rather than willful. Once a behavior is repeated it is learned. Behaviors followed by success or a reward or reinforcement are quickly learned. These learned behaviors are often strategies the child uses to cope with situations. Behaviors that are reinforced, allowed to continue, or not corrected will be repeated as long as the child is unaware that the behavior is inappropriate. When a child is confronted with a new situation, he responds with the behavior that now comes naturally.

Children often use similar strategies to cope with many different situations. They often learn and use only one or two different strategies, applying variations of them to adjust to different situations. Learned behaviors, or coping strategies, may be the only way the child knows to behave. After repeated use, the learned behavior becomes *established,* used over and over. Once a behavior is established, it may appear willful, as if the child is consciously using the behavior. It is important to realize that a child often acts without analyzing the behavior.

For example:

Jason is told it is bedtime. He screams, throws himself onto the floor and yells, "I don't want to go to bed!" Jason's behavior is a new, first-time response. If the next day he responds the same way when told to go to bed, the behavior may be learned. How his parents handle his behavior the first day may determine whether or not he repeats the behavior and if it becomes an established, learned behavior. Any response from the parents that reinforces the behavior will make it more likely to be repeated. Some responses include:

- Negative attention; for example, yelling at the child, getting angry or emotional.
- Success; for example, allowing him to stay up later.

A response that might extinguish the behavior, not reinforce it (therefore, not establish the tantrum as a learned behavior) would be quietly redirecting him to his feet, guiding him to bed, and ignoring his screaming.

Often, preventing a behavior from occurring or repeating is the best way to assure that a behavior is not learned. Once the behavior becomes established (used over and over), behavioral strategies must be used to effectively change the learned behavior.

Because a child uses similar learned behaviors to cope with different situations, it is important to know *why* the child is acting as he is. The focus needs to be on the *function* of the behavior rather than the actual behavior. In Jason's case the function of his behavior is both attention-seeking and avoidance of going to bed. Understanding the function of the behavior allows adults to teach the child more effective behaviors or coping strategies and to break the pattern of learned behaviors that are bothersome or that interfere with the child's ability to learn or function.

Is It Sensory?

Some children react to sensory input in a variety of ways. Inattention, distractibility, fidgeting, acting without thinking, and aggressive or defiant behaviors, such as pushing or striking out, all may have a sensory cause.

You might ask, "What do you mean by *sensory?*" There are sensory stimuli all around us, including vision (things we see), sounds, touch, smells, and movement. We experience external sensory input every day without thinking about it. We walk into a room that may be cluttered with things on the walls; there may be music playing in the background or a buzz from the fluorescent lights; we may pass the sweet smell of flowers or experience the movement of the car as we take a ride. We often take external sensory input for granted and do not think of how it can influence a person's behavior. Sensory input requires that the external environment interact with the child's internal environment or his body.

Some children have sensory processing difficulties that cause them to react differently to sensory input than others do. Their internal sensory environment is different from other children's, causing them to react with challenging or unusual behaviors to what appears to be nonthreatening sensory input. Their responses are due to their bodies' reactions to sensory input or sensory needs. Children's internal sensory environments may be *underresponsive*, making them ignore people or things around them or crave certain sensory input. Conversely, their internal sensory environment may be *overresponsive*, so that they avoid the sensory input.

Philippe is six years old. He just finished first grade. He is described as an anxious, fearful, and overly sensitive child. He has a fear of dogs, bike riding, and skating. He is picky about what he eats. The smallest thing can upset him. Disorder or any type of change easily annoys him. When he gets upset, he either cries uncontrollably or is furious and filled with rage; his tantrums can last for hours.

He is having difficulty socially. He doesn't fit in. He passionately loves basketball: playing it, watching it on TV, and going to games. However, he always has a meltdown when he goes to games; he is overwhelmed by the noise and smells. He has tried to join in neighborhood games, only to become furious over something that happened, cry uncontrollably with rage, and leave the game. He is described as a wimp, a crybaby, or spoiled. Other children make fun of him, have no tolerance for his behaviors, and feel it's not worth the aggravation to play with him. His mother cannot predict where or when something will upset him. She is frustrated to the point of not wanting to take him out in public for fear of his reactions and those of the people around him.

Philippe is smart, and thus far, his behavior hasn't affected his school performance. It breaks his parents' hearts to watch him struggle. They want to know if his behaviors are due to anxieties and a need to control everything. Is he sensory defensive and reacting to a need to control the sensory input? What can be done to help him? What should be done when he has a meltdown? Can it be prevented?

Philippe was referred to an occupational therapist for sensory integration therapy. His evaluation demonstrated postural control problems and hyperresponsiveness with defensiveness within the auditory, tactile, and vestibular systems. Because of his defensiveness, his coping strategy has been to control everyone and everything in his environment with his behaviors. His biggest fear is of animals because he cannot control them. He becomes extremely anxious in any situation that is new or that he cannot control. His anxiety and need for control is emotionally draining and exhausting for both him and his family.

Philippe works hard to control who touches him and when he is touched. He limits contact by people or animals and through activities he chooses. He loves physical activities and sports but cannot cope with the unexpected physical contact. He often reacts with hysterical crying or uncontrolled rage, striking out at those around him.

Sensory behaviors are provoked by the body's needs. If the sensory need is addressed, the behavior will often diminish. For Philippe, addressing his sensory defensiveness diminished many of his anxieties and controlling behaviors. It also improved his self-esteem and ability to interact with his peers.

A child confronted with a sensory situation may use one or two similar strategies to cope with many different situations. After repeated use, the behavior becomes learned and established. Philippe's coping strategy was to become angry, cry, and flee the situation. He used this strategy in every overwhelming sensory situation, and it worked for him. Many sensory behaviors, while triggered by the body's needs, may also be established behaviors that are learned, making them *both* sensory and behavior. The primary function of the behavior must be addressed first. For example, Philippe's sensory defensiveness must be addressed, and then the learned behavior can be dealt with by using behavioral techniques and teaching effective coping strategies.

Why Is It Important to Know the Difference?

Sensory processing disorders can be misconstrued as behavioral problems, inattention, distractibility, motor incoordination, hypersensitivity, or emotional difficulties. If we make the mistake of addressing only the behavioral aspect of the problem, the base sensory problem will still exist, and the child may become frustrated, act out in different or more intense ways, or project a feeling of uneasiness, as if something is about to erupt. Equally important is that when a sensory problem exists, it often is accompanied by behavioral concerns or coping strategies that also must be addressed. Atypical behaviors that are sensory in nature are often both behavioral and sensory. Excusing difficult behavior because it has a sensory foundation is a mistake. When dealing with sensory issues, we must make sure the underlying problem is not being overlooked (sensory) for what may be a quick fix (behavioral intervention). How we prioritize, coordinate, and implement our program becomes very important.

Philippe's occupational therapy program addressed both the behavioral and sensory issues. The program included strengthening his core postural muscles, improving his sensory integration and his self-esteem, and teaching him self-regulation strategies. Sensory activities were used in designing a sensory diet (see chapter 10) to aid him with self-regulation and emotional control.

Although the goal was to prevent meltdowns, there were times when they still occurred. Philippe was taught sensory strategies to regain control. As he improves in his ability to self-regulate and implement the strategies, the behaviors will be successfully prevented. Philippe's underlying problems are all sensory-related. However, the strategies he uses to cope are learned and difficult to change. Positive behavioral strategies are required to teach and motivate him to use new replacement behaviors.

Children are dynamic beings who are affected by and reflect things and people in their external environment and their internal state. They are also barometers of the emotional states of adults around them. Tasks and situations in which they feel threatened can trigger behavioral responses. The frustration experienced by teachers, parents, and therapists is fueled by the chaos witnessed in a child's behaviors. In analyzing the behavior, we realize that the problem is multifaceted and often has multiple causes. Thus, our approach must be multifaceted or nonlinear.

Chaos Theory

Behavioral problems in children are dynamic and complex, just as children are dynamic and complex. When we look at the behaviors, we are frequently confronted by what appears to be chaos. Chaos Theory was proposed to find order within dynamic, complex systems where unidirectional, linear solutions do not work.

Chaos Theory proposes that chaos is a form of order disguised as disorder (Coffey 1998). According to Royeen (2003), the theory suggests that even in cases of extreme disorder, what appears to be chaos actually has an underlying pattern or order. Similarly, we believe there is an underlying order to the complexities of and approach to addressing behaviors.

Royeen (2003) cites five key assumptions underlying chaotic systems. We believe these assumptions are directly applicable to behavior:

Interaction between and among variables is nonlinear.
So it is with behavior. Children's behaviors stem from interactions between sensory systems, the environment, people in the environment, task demands placed upon them, the state of their internal systems, and how they are feeling at any given moment. Each variable can affect the child's behavior inordinately one day and not at all on another.

Variables affect one another and are interdependent.
In life, all things are interrelated in some manner, but not in a linear relationship (Royeen 2003). The variables involved with behavior coexist and affect one another. A child who is tired or hungry may exhibit undesirable behaviors in a department store, demonstrating poor tolerance for noise levels, inability to wait quietly, or inability to interact well with others.

Chaotic systems exist in states of flux or turbulence, not in equilibrium.
Children who exhibit challenging or problematic behaviors often do so in response to changes or turbulence within themselves or their environment. When the forces within

the child and the environment are not equal (the edge of chaos), behavioral problems arise. When the forces inside the body are equal to the forces outside the body, chaos is never seen.

Chaotic systems are self-guided, self-organizing, and not hierarchical, and they demonstrate emergent behavior.

Children use behaviors to cope within their environments. Behaviors arise from a need, whether internal or external, and are the children's attempts to organize themselves, their world, and to function within it.

Chaotic systems possess an underlying order.

In spite of the apparent disorder associated with chaos, or the chaotic behaviors displayed by a child, there is an underlying order to what we see. The order is there, if we only know or understand the system that explains it. Our approach must be nonlinear because the system is nonlinear.

Children behave for specific reasons. There is order and purpose to what children do. Just as there are multiple forces in chaos, so are there multiple purposes served by most behaviors. Behaviors occur for multiple reasons and must be analyzed on many levels. Children are complex, changing beings. They react according to their physical and mental abilities, their emotional responses, and their sensory needs. *They also react by using learned responses.* A behavior may arise for one purpose and then be repeated for a different purpose or a learned result. Analyzing the problems within behavior, the primary cause, and the secondary reasons why behavior continues involves looking at multiple issues and requires applying a multidirectional approach.

Our Mission

As occupational and physical therapists, we deal with children who struggle with a myriad of disorders and difficulties. We have to deal with behaviors that are chaotic and overwhelming, and we are frequently asked by parents, teachers, and other caregivers to aid in identifying and altering problematic behaviors. Some of the questions frequently asked include:

- Is this child a bad child? Is he doing it willfully?

- My child is very controlling and manipulative. Is it sensory or is it behavior?

- How do I know if the behavior I am seeing is due to sensory integrative problems or to bad behavior?

- Everyone gives me advice about how to handle my child. Who do I listen to?

- Can a behavior be due to a sensory integrative problem and still be purposeful (behavioral)?

- How can I explain to others what my child is going through and how to handle and accept him?

- The behaviors are getting worse! We have done everything we can to change the behaviors and it didn't work. What do we do now?

- I know I am supposed to reward good behavior, but how can I just ignore all the bad behaviors?

The answers to these questions are not simple. There are many factors to consider for each behavior that arises. Questions like these were the impetus for writing this book.

Psychologists and behavioralists have addressed behavioral issues through functional behavioral analysis (FBA), applied behavioral analysis (ABA), and other behavioral techniques. In the last few decades the principles of ABA have been applied to patient populations that we, the authors, deal with in varying degrees of success. Because of the data accumulated during ABA, it is the most well documented and understood approach to addressing behavioral issues. Many behavioralists, psychologists, and physicians, however, still do not understand or may not acknowledge the influence of other factors, such as sensory processing, communication, and motor control, on behavior. Certainly these factors have not been explained in terms of dealing with behavioral intervention.

Our mission is to:

- Take known sensory-related behaviors and integrate them into traditionally accepted theories of behavioral analysis in order to look holistically at children, addressing both sensory and learned behaviors.

- Combine the two bodies of knowledge, sensory integration and behavioral intervention, to develop a comprehensive approach for dealing with problem behaviors.

- Develop an objective method to look at behaviors, identify the function of the behavior, and create a comprehensive intervention program.

- Focus on the critical thinking process and develop concrete indicators of when and how to implement specific strategies.

- Implement a user-friendly format by streamlining the analysis process, making order out of chaos, and succinctly identifying the needed intervention.

We have developed our mission statement to try to advocate for children who cannot identify their sensory processing or communication difficulties and also do not understand the impact these have on their behavior. Our goal is to help parents and caregivers develop a more holistic view and understanding of the child.

Our Philosophy

The premise of our approach and methodology revolves around these basic concepts:

1. Children have a fundamental need to function within their environment. All behaviors serve a function or purpose. Children often develop coping strategies or behaviors to help them function.

2. The child's behaviors are the result of:

   - The child trying to meet a specific need.

   - The child's response to an environmental demand or stimuli.

   - A learned response or a coping strategy.

3. Behaviors initially develop to meet a primary need (primary cause), and then they are maintained by the success encountered within their environment (primary and secondary reinforcers).

4. Behaviors are almost always maintained by more than one factor.

5. Behaviors that are repeated several times are *learned*. Behaviors that are used regularly are *established*.

6. Children can use the same behavior for many different reasons. The behaviors may look alike, but the causes may be very different.

7. Attitude is critical. You need to:

   ■ Believe that the child is capable of changing and overcoming his problems. Children have proven they can overcome anything.

   ■ Believe in your own abilities to change the child's behavior. If you believe you can, you can.

   ■ Be positive, supportive, and nonjudgmental.

8. Intervention must address the whole child: physically, mentally, emotionally, and sensory.

   ■ If a child views an activity as pleasurable, everything associated with it will be pleasurable.

   ■ You can't eliminate a behavior without teaching a replacement behavior. It is important to focus on what you want the child to be doing, not on what he or she is doing wrong.

Table 1.1
How This Book Will Help

This book is set up to give you the information you need to analyze any child's behavior, look at the function the behavior serves, prioritize goals, and implement an appropriate intervention.

Chapter 1, Is It Sensory or Is It Behavior?	Defines the importance of differentiating sensory from learned behaviors. We introduce the idea that the Chaos Theory can apply to behavior, and we explain our mission, our philosophy, and basic concepts important in understanding the causes of behaviors. This chapter provides the gateway to unraveling the mysteries of behavior.
Chapter 2, Sensory Integration and Sensory Processing Disorders	Provides a detailed description of the sensory systems, how they work, and how difficulties processing sensory information can affect behaviors. It provides a solid foundation for future chapters on analyzing behaviors.
Chapter 3, Deviations in Development: The Impact on Behavior	Briefly looks at both typical and atypical expressions in development and discusses how they affect behavior. This chapter does not contain an all-inclusive list, but does identify behaviors often noted by parents and others as problematic or worrisome.
Chapter 4, Basic Concepts: Analyzing Behaviors	Provides a detailed look at the ABC's of behavior (Antecedent, Behavior, and Consequences), describing the foundation skills needed to analyze, prioritize, and change behaviors.

(continued)

Table 1.1 How This Book Will Help (*Continued*)

Chapter 5, Sensory: Analyzing the Behavior	Objectively helps identify sensory-based behaviors, differentiating between sensory-obtaining and sensory-avoiding behaviors. Strategies to correct the underlying sensory problems are outlined.
Chapter 6, Analyzing Behaviors That Are Not Sensory	Discusses how learned behaviors result from the child's desire to obtain or avoid something. This chapter also looks at the reasons challenging behaviors occur and clearly outlines corrective action.
Chapter 7, Environmental Intervention Techniques	Looks at environmental modifications that can improve a child's performance and behavior. This chapter also discusses how behaviors can be altered just by changing the environment, thus saving time and energy for everyone involved.
Chapter 8, Behavioral Intervention Techniques	Provides concrete strategies to design and implement change whether the behaviors are sensory or learned.
Chapter 9, Handling Temper Tantrums and Challenging Behaviors	Helps objectify the unexpected, giving concrete strategies and guidelines for effectively handling tantrums.
Chapter 10, Sensory Diets	Looks at the key components of a sensory diet, which helps a child display appropriate levels of attention and focus, and powerful activities that can be used within your action plan.
Chapter 11, Case Study: Adam's School Behavior	Presents a case study of a seven-year-old with school-related problems. The chapter presents the ABC's of analyzing his behavior problems, objectively differentiating between sensory and non-sensory behaviors, defining and prioritizing the problematic behaviors and desired replacement behaviors, and identifying the most effective intervention.
Chapter 12, Case Study: Grace	Presents a case study of a three-and-a-half-year-old and describes her preschool experience, alluding to her skills, behaviors, and sensory difficulties. Using the Analyzing Behavior Worksheet, her behaviors are objectified into three clear problem behaviors with action plans that take into account learned behaviors, sensory concerns, and behavioral strategies.

Our Approach to Behavioral Intervention

We have introduced the concept of what is meant by sensory processing issues here, but will discuss the topic more fully in the ensuing chapters. When dealing with behavior problems, if sensory processing difficulties are not recognized or are ignored, the typical methods of behavioral intervention can produce disastrous outcomes. The child may become frustrated, self-injurious, or aggressive toward others, and those attempting to correct the original behaviors have inadvertently contributed to more alarming behaviors. The types of difficulties we see, as therapists trained in sensory integration, are outlined and described. Sensory integration, the process, is explained in chapter 2. The sensory systems are reviewed with descriptions of their functions and the difficulties or disorders within each of the systems. This information in chapter 2 is the foundation for understanding not only sensory integration and its relationship to behavior but also the information that follows in subsequent chapters.

Difficulties encountered by children with deviations in development are the basis for many of the behaviors that are worrisome to adults. Chapter 3 looks at the role of development in behavior. How a child learns to perceive his or her environment and interact within it is discussed. Behaviors that may be indicative of atypical development and the need for further medical investigation are also discussed. Although not meant to be an all-encompassing list, chapter 3 identifies behaviors that are often noted by parents as first indicators of an atypically developing child and problematic or worrisome behaviors.

Chapter 4 explains the ABC's of analyzing behavior, looking at the behavior (the B), what happened before the behavior (the A, or antecedent), and what came after the behavior (the C, or consequence). This approach looks at the phases of behavior. An understanding of this approach is required for analyzing, prioritizing, and changing the behavior. This information is critical to understanding ensuing chapters and using the methodology and worksheets provided later in the book.

In chapter 5 we tackle sensory-based behaviors with the goal of helping you to identify sensory behaviors, differentiating between those that are sensory-obtaining and sensory-avoiding. Because the interventions are different, the identification of the function of the behavior is critical to successfully changing the behavior. We have included strategies to correct the problems, based upon the identification of cause of the behavior.

Chapter 6 looks at behaviors that are not sensory-based. Here we look at normal behavioral issues that are seen on a regular basis with many children. These behavioral problems are often seen by themselves, or in combination with sensory issues. In the pursuit of trying to obtain or avoid, children quickly learn behaviors that will get them what they need. In this chapter we look at the reasons challenging behaviors occur and outline corrective action for dealing with the behaviors.

Environmental factors play a significant role in how a child behaves. Problematic behaviors can often be avoided or dealt with merely by changing the environment, thus avoiding the need to address the behavior and the chance of a negative interaction with the child. In chapter 7 we have included suggestions varying from flooring and lighting design to modifications as simple as alterations in task presentation. This chapter offers you choices of strategies that are feasible in any circumstance.

It is important to determine and focus on the behavior you want to see more than the behavior you want to get rid of. Chapter 8 helps you define desired behaviors and provides strategies to make these positive behaviors a reality. Your role and skill levels in dealing with behavior, developing and establishing new behaviors, the types and use of reinforcers, delaying gratification, and prompting the desired behavior are explained. Whether you are trying to replace ineffective behaviors caused by sensory or behavioral issues, this chapter gives concrete, specific methodologies to design and implement programs to alter worrisome behaviors.

Tantrums are frustrating and annoying, but they are a necessary part of dealing with children. All children utilize tantrums during development. Many will develop other coping strategies and skills that will negate the need to use tantrums to get what they need or want. Others need our help in doing so. Chapter 9 deals with tantrums, giving you the objectivity and methods to guide the child to more productive methods of interaction, whether the underlying problem is sensory or behavioral.

Sensory diets are discussed in chapter 10. These useful strategies can aid in regulating the child's attention, arousal, focus, and effort. Behavioral control and regulation is the goal and sensory diets, the tools. However, in order to be effective, sensory diets must be individualized, focused applications, and not applied in a shotgun approach with scattered use and effectiveness. The *what, how,* and *when* to use sensory diets are discussed.

Finally, in order to integrate all of this information, we have provided two case studies in chapters 11 and 12. We have chosen a boy with school-related problems and a girl in her preschool years. We describe the worrisome behaviors and take you through our process of behavioral analysis. We include problem identification, prioritization, and identification of desired replacement behaviors; differentiate sensory and non-sensory-based behavior; and outline sensory diets and the interventions that have proven successful. The Analyzing Behavior Worksheet in appendix D will aid you through the process of behavioral interventions.

Sensory Integration and Sensory Processing Disorders 2

Children with sensory integrative difficulties are not easy to understand or deal with. They may appear overly sensitive, explosive, picky, inflexible, controlling, or rude. They may be uncoordinated and clumsy. They may become either clingy or standoffish and demanding in order to organize the quantity and type of sensory input that bombards them. They may withdraw or push people away because they are threatened by uninvited touch. They may not accept being cuddled by their family members. They may demand certain articles of clothing or food, while refusing others. They often cannot verbalize the cause of their problems. They don't know what is wrong and often do not know why they behave the way they do.

Parents, teachers, therapists, and professionals struggle to make sense of these behaviors. In their attempts to make order out of disorder, they attribute the causes for the behaviors to the child's temperament or personality, environmental demands or lack of demands, the child's lack of knowledge of appropriate behavior, or the parents' poor parenting skills. The children are often labeled as spoiled, shy, headstrong, stubborn, or lazy. The behaviors may be attributed to the child's personality or discounted as normal for his age. Such simplifications of the problem behaviors can be frustrating to both parents and professionals who believe in their hearts that these behaviors have another cause.

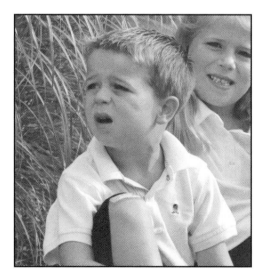

What appears to be behavioral (tantrums, stubbornness, or over-reacting) may be sensory-related.

Traditional behavioral approaches and positive reward systems may be partially successful, but behaviors continue to be problematic or worrisome. Parents report that sensory-based problems occur across multiple environments and situations. When purely behavioral strategies are used with children with sensory-based behaviors, they do not treat the entire problem, and therefore, are only partially successful.

The mystery behind the myriad of unusual or confusing behaviors displayed by many children can often be unraveled through understanding the sensory systems and the role sensory integration has in normal development. It is through understanding sensory integrative dysfunction and how it relates to a child's behavior that we can give order to the chaos of behaviors we observe and develop a comprehensive program to address the problem.

Sensory Integration

What is Sensory Integration?

Sensory integration (SI) is a theory and technique developed by A. Jean Ayres, a psychologist and occupational therapist. Her career was devoted to the organization, development, and testing of her theories. She began her work in SI during her postdoctoral studies at the National Institute of Child Development at the Center for Health Sciences at the University of California in Los Angeles in the 1960s. Her work spanned the next three decades.

Initially Ayres' interest and research focused on the impact of visual perception and motor control on learning. She quickly expanded her research to include the other sensory systems, including the vestibular, proprioceptive, and tactile systems. Ayres postulated that sensory processing could have a direct impact on a child's ability to learn and perform. She developed standardized tests to measure the visual, vestibular, tactile, and proprioceptive systems. The test measures were combined with clinical observation of muscle tone, postural control, and balance as further measures of neuromotor maturation. Factor analytic studies were then completed to analyze patterns of dysfunction among learning disabled children. Through these factor analytic studies, Ayres identified dysfunctions in sensory processing of tactile, vestibular, proprioceptive, and visual systems that interfere with motor planning, language, behavior, cognition, and emotional well-being. The theory of sensory integration evolved as a direct result of Ayres' interpretation of this data.

Sensory integration, simply put, is the ability to take in information through our senses (touch, movement, smell, taste, vision, and hearing), put it together with prior information, memories, and knowledge stored in the brain, and make a meaningful response. It is a nonlinear process that is dependent upon the efficient integration of all the sensory experiences mixed with the environmental situations and demands and the child's own personality and reactions. Normal sensory integration allows the child to interact appropriately within his environment.

In the normally developing child, sensory integration occurs when the child participates in everyday activities. The child's love for sensory activities fuels an inner drive and motivation to conquer challenges. That drive urges the child to participate actively in experiences that promote sensory integration: The child explores the environment, tries new activities, and strives to meet increasingly more complex challenges. Mastering new challenges makes the child feel successful and gives him the confidence to try more difficult tasks.

Sensory integration occurs in the central nervous system (CNS) and is a neurological process that happens with little conscious attention or effort. The process is multifaceted and very complex. It requires the integration of external and internal information within the brain and the ability to use this information functionally through appropriate adaptive responses.

Sensory integration is believed to take place in the midbrain and brainstem levels in complex interactions with the parts of the brain that are responsible for development: coordination, attention, arousal levels, autonomic functioning, emotions, memory, and higher-level cognitive functions. Ayres and her followers believe the process of sensory integration forms a crucial foundation for later, more complex learning and behavior (Ayres 1979).

Sensory integration should never be mistaken for sensory stimulation. Sensory stimulation involves using sensory input for the pure sake of the sensory input. No demand is placed on the individual, and therefore no "integration" is needed within the brain. An example of sensory stimulation might be a massage; spinning; or playing in shaving cream, sand, a rice box, or a ball pool. The child enjoys playing in the various textures but is not asked to integrate the information for a meaningful response. For sensory integration to occur the child must interact adaptively with the sensory medium in a challenging way. For example, playing in a rice box or ball pool is sensory stimulation, while feeling for small objects hidden under the sand or balls would require "integration" of the senses.

The Senses

The sensations that the nervous system recognizes are touch, sight, hearing, smell, taste, and the "hidden senses." The hidden senses relate to body position (proprioception) and movement (vestibular) (Haron 1999).

Tactile or Touch

Touch, or the tactile sense, is located in the skin and mouth. Its influences are pervasive, and it affects how we see our world. By processing touch information, we feel safe, which allows us to bond with others and develop socially and emotionally. The tactile system comprises the discriminatory and protective systems. The discriminatory system allows us to determine what we are touching and to define the spatial characteristics of objects. Moreover, it tells us when and where we are touched. The protective system tells us when we are in contact with something dangerous or threatening. It causes a fright, flight, or fight response, which involves the whole mind and body. It is the protective system that activates when we are walking alone at night down a dark road and we feel a light touch on our back.

Proprioception

Body position sense, or the proprioceptive sense, is located in our muscles and joints. It is an unconscious sense that detects where our body parts are in space and how they are moving. Proprioceptive information gives us a clear map of how our body is put together. It defines our internal body awareness and allows us to appreciate how our body relates to the external environment. It tells us how hard we are pushing or touching things and allows us to gauge how much pressure we need to perform any given task. It is the system through which we perceive touch or pressure and resistance to movement, as well as the calming effect of those two sensations. The proprioceptive system perceives the benefits of a massage or heavy exercise and can be used for calming and organizing a child.

Proprioception is defined as the cornerstone of sensory integrative intervention (Roley, Blanche, and Shaaf 2001). Its input has the capacity to affect arousal levels, specifically by calming and organizing a person who is overstimulated. It also exerts a regulatory influence over other sensory systems, helping to calm and organize the nervous system when overresponding to tactile (touch) or vestibular (movement) sensations. Activities rich in proprioception are key components to sensory integrative intervention programs because they can help increase the feedback a child receives from his motor movements, improve body awareness, normalize arousal levels, and aid in self-regulation.

Proprioception results from joint traction, compression, or resistance to movement, which occurs during heavy work or play sessions when weights are used or when children use their own body weight as resistance. Examples include climbing on playground equipment, such as monkey bars, ladders, ropes, or walls; wheelbarrow walking; or tug-of-war games.

Vestibular

The sense of movement, or vestibular sense, detects our head movements relative to gravity. Vestibular sensory receptors, located in the inner ear, provide information about gravity, balance, and movement. The vestibular sense tells us whether or not we are moving, how quickly, and in what direction. It provides us with the sense of safety that can come only from knowing our feet are planted firmly on the ground. It also gives us a physical reference that can help us make sense of visual information, particularly where we are in relationship to other things in our environment, and how other objects relate to each other (Trott, Laurel, and Windeck 1993). Vestibular input contributes to our sense of balance, head control, eye gaze, coordination of the two sides of the body, muscle tone, and posture and contributes to a child having core stability both physically and emotionally.

The vestibular system has the power to influence our nervous system and has a direct impact on our arousal. Fast movements tend to wake us up, while slow rhythmic movements put us to sleep. Linear, straight-up-and-down, or forward and backward movements, such as jumping on a trampoline or riding in a car, tend to be organizing, while rotary movements such as spinning or turning in a circle can have an alerting and sometimes disorganizing effect.

Integration of Senses

The senses never work in isolation. Each sense works with the others to form a composite picture of who we are, where we are, and what is going on around us. Sensory integration is crucial in producing this composite picture. The sensory information enters the nervous system and is integrated with other sensory, environmental, and experiential information. For example:

- Tactile information integrates with visual perception. As children learn the spatial qualities of an object through touch, they connect it to the visual image they perceive, learning visual-spatial concepts that will eventually be important for reading and writing.

- Tactile combines with proprioceptive information (touch receptors and joint receptors) to help children discern their movements and relationship to other objects. The combination of these senses allows children to identify with their fingers objects hidden deep in their pockets and to exert the appropriate pressure to avoid breaking toys or tearing the paper when writing. This combination also tells us unconsciously how our tongue is moving to articulate sounds.

- Vestibular combines with proprioceptive and tactile information to give children a good body scheme and awareness of how they are moving through space. It provides a foundation that allows the child to move in a smooth, coordinated fashion.

Sensory Processing Disorders

Sensory processing disorders (SPD), also known as sensory integrative dysfunction, dysfunction of sensory integration (DSI), sensory integrative dysfunction, and SI dysfunction, occur when the brain is not able to organize sensory information. Either the senses are delivering information that may not be accurate or, once the information gets into the system, the interconnections within the brain are not efficient and the information is not processed accurately.

Ayres (1979) described sensory integration with an analogy comparing the brain to a large city with traffic consisting of neural impulses. Good sensory processing enables all the impulses to flow easily and reach their destinations quickly. Sensory integrative dysfunction, on the other hand, causes a traffic jam in the brain. Some sensory information gets tied up in the traffic, blocking certain parts of the brain from getting the information they need to do their job. According to Ayres, "When the flow of sensation is disorganized, life can be a rush-hour traffic jam" (1979, p. 51).

The hallmarks of sensory integrative dysfunction are inconsistencies in performance; difficulties in attention, arousal, organization of behaviors, motor planning, and coordination; difficulties processing; and fluctuations in emotions and behavior. SI dysfunction is a central processing disorder or a disorder in the normal neurological process. At certain times of the day the traffic may not flow well; there may be an accident, and traffic may be diverted to alternate routes; or it may just stop. A traffic jam causes a breakdown in efficiency, and frequently emotions flair. When the brain is not processing sensory input well, it is usually not directing behavior or emotions effectively. The child with a sensory integration disorder cannot respond to sensory information in a consistent, meaningful way. Without good sensory integration, learning is difficult; the child cannot cope with ordinary demands, which may lead to poor self-esteem.

It is estimated that twelve to thirty percent of all children have SI problems (Haron 1999). Sensory integrative disorders can occur in children who have no medical diagnoses. "Normal" children are frequently challenged by inefficient sensory integration to such a degree that they seek help and intervention. These children have no identified disabilities and appear to be gifted with good health, intelligence, and strong, loving families, yet they struggle with the challenges of everyday living. They have difficulties regulating their attention and activity levels, planning and organizing their motor actions, or tolerating ordinary sensations. Because the inefficiencies in sensory processing negatively affect their skill development, they have to work harder than other children at some tasks. Coping with stress or change, sharing with others, paying attention, or even sitting still may be difficult for them.

Frequently, SI dysfunction coexists with other diagnoses, such as learning disabilities and attention deficits. According to Mulligan (2003), research shows that specific patterns of disorders of sensory integration exist in children diagnosed with attention deficit, learning disabilities, developmental delays, autism, and fragile X syndrome. Also at high risk for disorders of sensory integration are low-birth-weight infants and postinstitutional children.

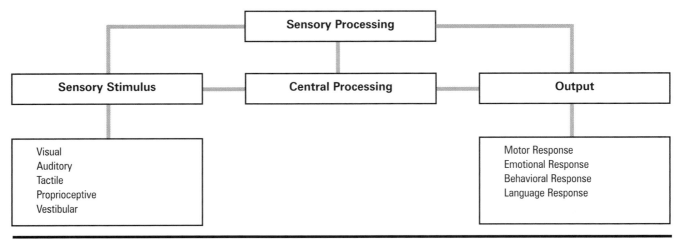

Figure 2.1   Three phases of sensory processing

Identifying Sensory Processing Disorders

Sensory processing dysfunctions can occur because of a breakdown in any of the three phases of sensory integration: taking information in through our senses (sensory stimulus), putting it together with other information (central processing), or making a meaningful motor, language, behavioral, or emotional response (output). Because sensory integration involves all three steps, it is nearly impossible to separate these functions. Once the sensory input streams into the nervous system, it is relayed to other parts of the brain and immediately involves central processing. It is a nonlinear process that is explained here in simple linear terms.

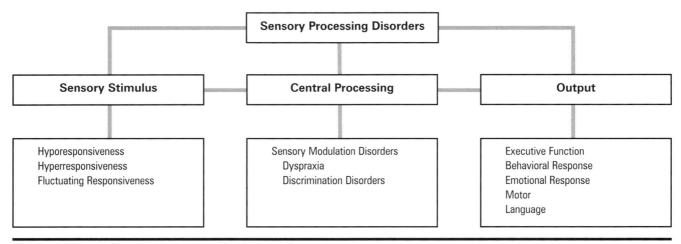

Figure 2.2   Sensory processing disorders

Sensory Stimulus Dysfunctions

Children with sensory integrative dysfunction may not respond to sensory information the way other children do. They may be hypersensitive, hyposensitive, or fluctuate in their responses. They may also respond differently based on their responsivity and the sensory system involved.

Sensory Hypersensitivity

Hypersensitivity, also known as hyperresponsiveness or oversensitivity, is characterized by avoidance behaviors to sensory activities or situations. The brain of the hypersensitive child registers sensations too intensely. Emotionally charged behaviors, characterized by fright, flight, or fight, are frequently seen as the child misinterprets normal sensory input as life-threatening intrusions requiring the child to either become immobilized by fear, run, or defend himself. The hypersensitive child may react to a small bruise as if it were a broken arm, a casual touch as a blow, or a stumble as a fall from the roof. Emotionally charged avoidance behaviors may include fleeing the area, being irritated or annoyed, and appearing threatened or aggressive toward others. The child may react to the slightest touch or movement with increased anxiety, hostility, or even defensive behaviors. He or she will avoid situations or activities that are viewed as threatening or may also rely on routine, predictable activities to keep his anxieties in control. Because of this, the child may react negatively to changes in routine. Distractibility and emotional hypersensitivity are common as the child goes into defensive mode, pays attention to all stimuli, and is keenly aware of other people's actions.

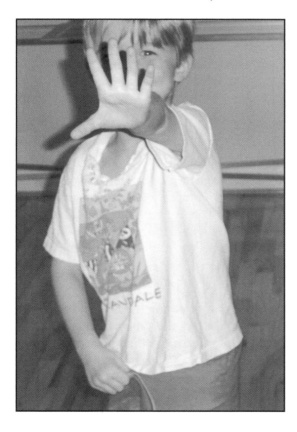

A child with hypersensitivities may be threatened and react defensively to normal stimuli.

The hypersensitive child may also "shut down." A child who runs to a corner, hides under a desk, or becomes passive and lethargic may have reached his saturation point for sensory input and shut down to avoid interacting.

The sensory systems that are hypersensitive will affect the type of behavioral responses a child will make. The child who has auditory hypersensitivity may avoid or react to crowded or noisy rooms such as restaurants, cafeterias, auditoriums, or places with loud music. The child with tactile defensiveness may avoid certain textures in clothing, food, haircuts, or baths. He may also avoid crowded environments for fear of being touched or bumped without warning, as opposed to the child who reacts to the noise in the environment. A child with vestibular hypersensitivities will react to changes in position or to the possibility of being moved. The child may refuse to lie on his back or stomach, avoid riding a bicycle, using skates, playing at playgrounds, or just walking down a street or up a hill. The defensive child may complain of feeling ill, get carsick, or complain of headaches or stomachaches. A checklist of common behaviors can be found in appendix B.

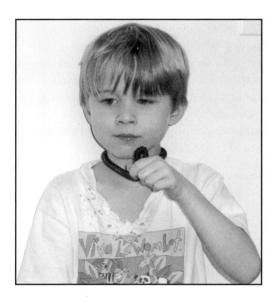

A child who is stressed or under-responsive may mouth objects or his shirt. Here a chewy is used to substitute for his shirt.

Sensory Hyposensitivity

Sensory-seeking or obtaining behaviors characterize hyposensitivity, also known as hyporesponsiveness or undersensitivity. The brain of the hyposensitive child registers sensations less intensely than those of others. The hyposensitive child does not get sufficient sensory information and requires more stimulation than other children to elicit similar responses. The child may demonstrate two different sets of behaviors: either sensory-seeking or passive with poor registration.

Sensory-Seeking

The sensory-seeking child will actively seek out or obtain the needed sensory input. The sensory system that is underresponsive will affect the type of behavioral responses a child will make. Children that are underresponsive within the tactile system will be "touchy-feely," touching everything in sight. They may take things from other children, or mouth objects or their shirts. These children may frequently bump into people and objects; they may be a safety hazard and be unaware of impending danger. Their high activity level, driven by sensory needs, combined with dulled awareness of the environment, creates situations that are an accident waiting to happen. Missing cues other children pick up easily, sensory-seeking children won't notice that something is hot, sharp, or breakable. In addition, they may not notice when they injure themselves, as their threshold for registering sensory input is very high. Children who fluctuate in their responsivity may at other times react to the sight of an injury by crying and running to mother. Once consoled, they go on to the next activity, forgetting they were ever injured.

These children have such a high threshold for registering sensory information that they do not receive adequate information from their hands, legs, and mouth. They must repeatedly touch and feel objects (or mouth objects) to learn about their weight, texture, and shape. This inability to use touch information discriminately is a system or central processing problem called tactile discrimination disorder.

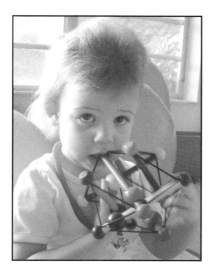

A child with a high threshold for registering sensory information (underresponsive) often mouths objects to gain more sensory information about the object.

Tactile discrimination disorder interferes with the child's ability to perform skilled discriminatory tasks. Children with this disorder may have difficulty isolating their fingers to show how old they are; holding and controlling a pencil or utensil; writing without looking at their fingers; articulating sounds; or blowing whistles. Their gross motor skills are often awkward and uncoordinated, and they may have difficulty with age-appropriate skills, such as riding a bike, skating, and other sports activities. Refer to appendix A for more characteristics.

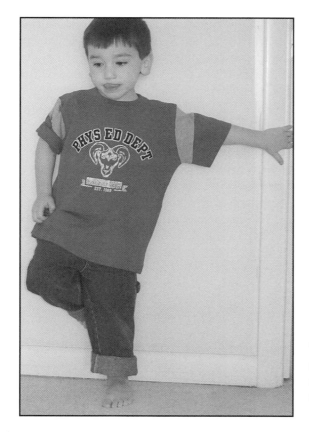

Tactile discrimination disorders affect gross motor skills, making a child awkward and uncoordinated.

Children who are hyposensitive within the proprioceptive system may demonstrate the above characteristics. In addition, they will have difficulty knowing how much pressure to exert with their arms and legs. They may push too hard, breaking toys or the lead of pencils when writing. They may press too lightly for their writing to be read. Gross motor skills appear awkward and uncoordinated. Body awareness and motor planning difficulties may make them appear awkward or may cause them to bump into things or trip for no apparent reason. They may be timid in new situations, lack self-confidence, and resist new physical challenges. Emotionally, they may be afraid of the dark and may demonstrate a rigid adherence to familiar activities.

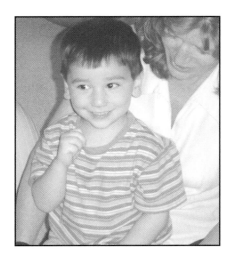 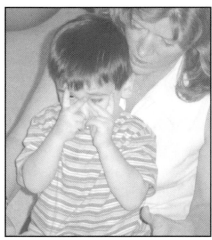 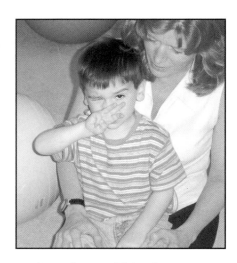

The child may have difficulty isolating his fingers to show how old he is.

Children who are hyposensitive within the vestibular system will seek out additional movement. They may have difficulty staying in their seat or sitting still. They may jump up and down, rock, or crave intense movement experiences. They may love being thrown in the air, assume an upside-down position, spin continually, or jump on a trampoline. They may be thrill seekers, enjoying fast-moving or scary rides; they may dart from one activity to another, moving fast to take advantage of momentum. Moving fast requires less control and energy than moving slowly.

Other children with the same issue will find their body loose and floppy. They may tire easily, slouch, and not have enough energy to move. They will have balance or coordination problems. Coordinating the two sides of their body may be difficult, and they may not have consistent hand dominance. Eye movements may also be affected. They may have difficulty with gaze stability, eye control, and visual perception. These children may also demonstrate a hyporesponsive auditory system, with auditory processing and discrimination difficulties.

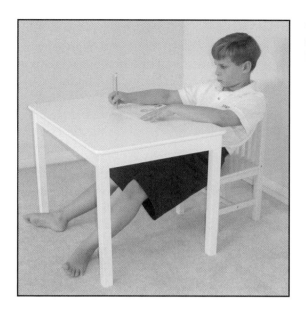

Children who are underresponsive may have difficulty staying in their seat or sitting still.

Passive With Poor Registration

The hyposensitive child may also present as a passive child with poor registration, rather than sensory-seeking. The passive child accepts the decreased sensory input of hyposensitivity as normal and functions within a state of sensory deprivation. The sensory stimuli is perceived as insignificant by the nervous system and disregarded, resulting in the child not registering the information. The child is a passive participant in the environment rather than being active, self-motivated, and exploring. If the vestibular system is involved, he may also have low muscle tone (floppy muscles), have low endurance, and be described as lazy or a couch potato. This decreased environmental interaction can have a negative effect on learning.

A checklist of common behaviors can be found in appendix A.

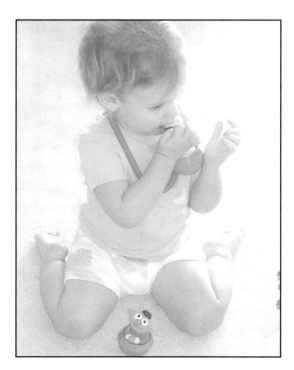

A child who is underresponsive to vestibular input may collapse to the floor. A W-sit posture is frequently used by children with low muscle tone.

Fluctuating Responses/Sensitivities

Children with fluctuating responses, a combination of hyper and hypo sensitivities, will display both sets of behaviors. This is seen frequently. Their nervous systems are in flux and have difficulty modulating and regulating the sensory input. The traffic in the brain either backs up (hyposensitive) or rushes through (hypersensitive). A child may crave intense crashing and hugging while at the same time not tolerating the tag in his shirt or the seams in his socks. How the child responds may depend on the time of the day, the place, or the type of stimuli.

Hypersensitivity and hyposensitivity, while characterized by either sensory-avoiding (escape) or sensory-seeking (obtaining) behaviors, share common threads. They are both characterized by inefficient processing of sensory stimuli. In the hypersensitive child, too much information gets in and the child avoids it, while in the hyposensitive child, too little information gets in. This state of sensory deprivation results in unpredictable behaviors characterized by both sensory-seeking and avoiding behaviors.

When a child demonstrates fluctuating responses, it is important to analyze whether the majority of the behaviors appear hypo- or hypersensitive to sensory input. Intervention should target the most consistent responses. If it's too hard to tell, intervention should cautiously follow the protocol for hypersensitivity.

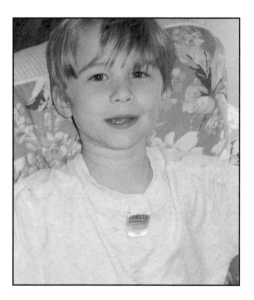

A child who fluctuates may show signs of both under- and overresponsiveness, not noticing food on his face while being unable to tolerate the tag on his shirt.

Central Processing Disorders

Sensory processing dysfunction occurs when the brain is unable to organize sensory information for use, causing a disruption between the sensory input and the motor output. Either the sensory information coming in is not accurate (sensory stimulus disturbance) or the input is not efficiently interconnected within the brain, so the child may have difficulty putting together the information from various senses (central processing). It is as if the brain is not connecting what is heard, with what is being seen, with how the child is moving. Experiences may lack meaning or be distorted. Without good sensorimotor experiences that are meaningful, the child may not develop the foundation skills necessary for building more advanced skills (Murray-Slutsky and Paris 2000).

Central processing disorders occur when children have difficulty combining sensory input with other information to make a meaningful response. Bundy, Lane, and Murray (2002) believe SI dysfunction manifests itself in two major ways: poor modulation and poor praxis. Individuals are not restricted to demonstrating one or the other type of dysfunction, but may show a combination of symptoms.

Sensory Modulation and Self-Regulation

Sensory modulation refers to the ability of the nervous system to regulate, organize, and prioritize incoming sensory information, inhibiting or suppressing irrelevant information and helping the child focus on relevant information. A well-modulated nervous system adapts to changes in the environment, has a level of arousal and attention appropriate for the task, blocks out irrelevant information, attends to relevant stimulation, and responds appropriately and in direct proportion to the input (Murray-Slutsky and Paris 2000).

Sensory *modulation* results in appropriate:

- Registration,
- Arousal,
- Self-regulation,
- Attention,
- Focus, and
- Behavior or emotional responses.

Sensory *registration* is the process by which children respond or attend to sensory input in their environment. The nervous system must first notice the sensory information. After it is registered, children check their memories to compare it to things they have heard or seen before, and thus give the new information meaning. They will then either arouse to the sensory input and prepare for action or move on. Children who fail to respond or have delayed responses to sensory information have diminished sensory registration. Examples include failing to respond when their names are called, not noticing a new toy, or being oblivious to other people in the room. Diminished sensory registration is often associated with one or two weaker sensory systems, such as the auditory or vestibular system. Without sensory registration, no other learning can take place.

Arousal describes how alert one feels. To attend, concentrate, and perform tasks in a manner suitable to the situational demands, one's nervous system must be in an optimal state of arousal for a particular task (Mercer and Snell 1977). Everyone has individual variations in their resting arousal level. Some people always appear to be operating in high gear, constantly moving and on the go, while others seem to be in low gear, moving slowly, appearing lethargic, and having difficulty finishing their work. Throughout the day our level of arousal increases and decreases. Our environment affects it both internally and externally. If you are hungry, your blood sugar may drop, lowering your arousal level internally. External events, such as a loud, crowded auditorium or cafeteria, children arguing, a fire bell going off, loud music, or TV, can quickly increase arousal levels.

Self-regulation is the ability to attain, maintain, and change the arousal level appropriate for a task or situation. Throughout each day we try to adjust our level of arousal according to each activity. We have learned tricks that work for increasing or decreasing our arousal level depending on the activity. For example, in the morning you may wake up tired and underaroused. A hot or cold shower, cup of coffee, or a morning exercise ritual may be all you need to raise your arousal level to handle the day. Each of us has an *optimal level of arousal* in which we function best. This optimal level may change based on the activity we are asked to do. For example, the optimal level of arousal needed for sitting at a desk reviewing numbers or working on a computer would be different than the level you need to make a presentation to your boss and the board of directors. To change your level of arousal you may use oral, vestibular, proprioceptive, tactile, visual, or auditory stimuli without ever realizing that you are using them. You may put something with a crunchy texture in your mouth to wake you up or suck hard candies to relax you; choose to move by exercising, rocking, tapping your foot or hand; fidget; look at something quieting or relaxing; or listen to music. The end result is the optimal level of arousal.

The *calm-alert state* is a window in which our ability to function is maximized. It is the optimal level of arousal for learning. In this state, we have a balance between the ability to attend to a stimulus or task and the level of arousal within our brains and bodies to prepare us to respond. We all need a certain amount of stress or stimulation to bring our levels of attention and arousal to optimum levels. If we lack that level of stimulation, our systems are sluggish and hyporesponsive. We may not register easily, have difficulty allocating our attention to the task, and be unable to process or assimilate information well. Similarly, if our systems are overaroused or overstimulated, we are not able to process or assimilate information. We may be hyperresponsive and overregistering to multiple stimuli and have difficulty filtering out pertinent from nonpertinent information. In the calm-alert state, we have sufficient levels of stimulation to be open to learning, processing, or functioning, yet not to the point at which stimulation begins to interfere (Murray-Slutsky and Paris 2000).

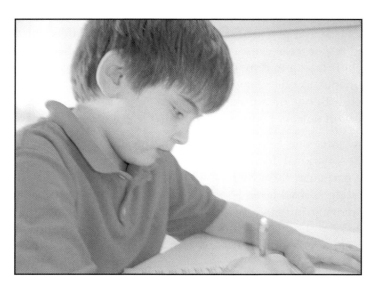

The "calm-alert state" is a window in which our ability to function is maximized.

Disorders of Sensory Regulation or Modulation

Sensory modulation disorder refers to a problem in the capacity to regulate and organize the degree, intensity, and nature of response to sensory input in a graded and adaptive manner. It is the inability to effectively regulate arousal levels or match the arousal level to the activity. A modulation disorder interferes with a person's ability to maintain an optimal level of arousal appropriate for the task, and therefore, interferes with a person's ability to effectively meet the challenges encountered every day.

A child or adult with a modulation disorder would display difficulties in several of the following: adapting to changes in the environment, responding in an organized fashion, using a level of arousal and attention appropriate for the task, blocking out irrelevant information, attending to relevant stimulation, and responding appropriately and in direct proportion to the input.

Sensory modulation disorders are characterized by difficulty with:

- Registration
- Attention
- Focus
- Arousal
  - Overarousal
  - Underarousal
  - Fluctuating arousal
- Self-regulation
- Behavior or emotional responses

Arousal levels of children or adults with a modulation disorder are often inappropriate. Children must find the *middle ground* and the appropriate level of arousal to allow them to interact effectively. Instead of finding middle ground, children with modulation disorders over- or under-respond to sensory input. The resulting behavior reflects a cascade of events within the central nervous system that affect attention, arousal, emotional stability, and cognitive processing (Bundy, Lane, and Murray 2002). Children having difficulty maintaining the middle ground may display one or all of the following problems:

- Resting arousal level is too high or too low.
- An inability to find, recognize, or maintain the middle ground appropriate for the task.
- Sensory processing deficits (over-, under-, or fluctuating responses to sensory input).

They may consistently be starting out in high gear and unable to slow down. With a high resting arousal level, they may quickly overstimulate with little provocation. They may be described as emotionally reactive, distractible, inattentive, aggressive, or anxious. They may flee or run from situations and people. Starting at the high end of middle ground, they may not be able to quickly or easily lower their thresholds and regain their composures. If the problem is due to inefficient processing of sensory stimuli (oversensitivity), the emotional and behavioral reactions may be characterized by fright, flight, or fight, or the child may shut down.

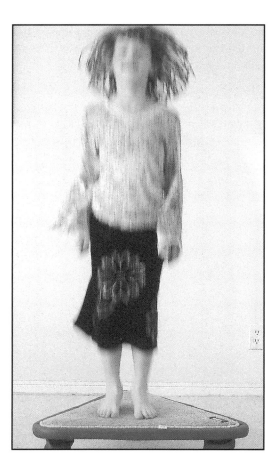

The child who is in constant motion may have difficulty finding and maintaining middle ground appropriate to the task.

Children with modulation disorders may also consistently be starting out in low gear and unable to wake up their system. They may have low muscle tone, lack facial and emotional expression, be oblivious to things around them, have difficulty registering aspects of their environment, slouch or fall out of a chair, choose sedentary activities, and appear sluggish. They may be described as a couch potato, lazy, passive, or as having low endurance. Starting at the low end of middle ground, it takes a lot of effort to get them up to a functional level of arousal. If the problem is due to inefficient processing of sensory stimuli (undersensitivity) these children may exert a great deal of effort to increase their arousal levels. Muscular efforts may be difficult. The child may simply avoid play or other activities because they are too difficult. When the child does make an effort, it may be characterized as all-or-none with poor grading of the activity. These children may constantly be on the go, running from thing to thing, and be described as inattentive or distractible with poor overall awareness. When they stop, they may fall asleep.

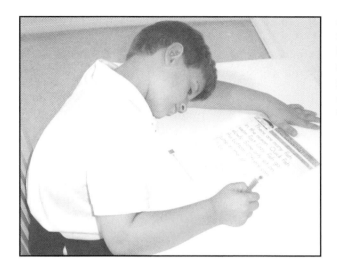

A child with poor sensory modulation, operating in low gear or underresponsive, will have difficulty generating enough muscle effort and may collapse to the table when writing.

Bundy, Lane, and Murray (2002) identify four common sensory modulation disorders. They include one sensory seeking or obtaining behavior called underresponsiveness to sensory input, and three characterized by avoidance behaviors or hypersensitivities: sensory defensiveness, gravitational insecurity, and aversive response to movement. Each of the common modulation disorders manifests differently depending on the sensory system most affected and whether the child is under- or oversensitive. Sensory defensiveness (hypersensitivities to sensory input) can occur in any of the sensory systems and frequently elicits the avoidance behaviors characterized by fright, flight, or fight. Tactile defensiveness, avoidance of normal tactile sensory experiences, is the most common form of defensiveness. Fear of movement, hypersensitivity, and poor processing of vestibular input characterize gravitational insecurity and aversive response to movement.

Stress and anxiety negatively affect sensory modulation. They move the child out of the calm-alert state by increasing arousal levels and have a negative impact on learning, skill acquisition, and overall function. Children who are underresponsive to sensory input (sensory-seeking or obtaining) may find that a slight increase in arousal helps them function, yet too much puts them outside the optimal level required to attend to a task. The child who is hypersensitive to sensory input (sensory-avoiding) is already operating at the high end of arousal. Stress and anxiety bump the arousal level outside the functional range. They interfere with the ability to filter out unimportant information; block sensory registration; amplify sensory defensiveness or sensory hypersensitivity; and increase distractibility, restlessness, and concentration difficulties. Interestingly, stress and anxiety provoke the same physiological response whether or not the threat is real. If the child perceives the situation to be stressful, he will react accordingly.

Gray (1982) described *behavioral inhibition* and its association with anxiety. He believed that if the experience matches what the child expects, then the child's behavior continues uninterrupted. However, if the experience does not match the expectation, then the behavior is interrupted (inhibited), anxiety and arousal increase, and the child pays close attention to all incoming stimuli. Anxiety, sensory defensiveness, attention to irrelevant sensory input, alterations in sensory registration, and modulation difficulties can ensue. Conversely, if the child knows what to expect, has positive memories of associated events, and experiences what he believes will occur, then anxiety is reduced and the behavior will continue uninterrupted. Structure during change, reviewing what to expect prior to novel situations, controlling environmental factors for maximum predictability, and assuring good open communication are pivotal to decreasing stress and anxiety and helping the child function automatically. Refer to chapter 7, Environmental Intervention Techniques, and Table 4.1 for more information.

Children with arousal levels that are inappropriately high or low may choose not to do the things that are most helpful. Children who need to move may not be motivated to move, just as children who need a physical outlet may not instinctively know what to do or how to use their time effectively. These children often come in from playtime more disorganized than they went out. Exercise, recess, and playtimes may need to be structured to allow the child opportunities to work on sensory processing and self-regulation. It is important to schedule sensory motor activities throughout the child's day, at school and at home, to ensure that the child engages in helpful activities. Recess may need to have structured games; the child may be limited to certain areas or activities or given a specific set of exercises or activities to complete.

Learned responses play a role in modulation disorders. We all base our expectations on past events and experiences. When we anticipate an uncomfortable or aggravating situation, stress and anxiety increase and avoidance behaviors follow. A child who is hypersensitive to sensory input may display avoidance behaviors long after the sensory input is no longer noxious to the nervous system. Memories of painful, unpleasant experiences remain to fuel the child's behavior. To unlearn the response (behavior), a child must understand (physically, emotionally, and cognitively) that the sensory input is not offensive or threatening.

Praxis

Children look at toys and objects creatively, inventing many ingenious ways to play with them. They coordinate their movements to catch a ball, skip, and excel at sports that require advanced timing and sequencing of motor movements. When they run into a problem they come up with innovative solutions and work on it until it's solved. These activities require *praxis,* or motor planning. Praxis is the ability to plan, organize, and carry out a sequence of unfamiliar actions. It is central to learning and requires the child to receive, process, and coordinate sensory information from his senses. When accurate sensory information comes into the child's nervous system, it forms a solid foundation for body scheme and body movements from which more advanced skills can be built.

Fundamental to praxis is sensory processing. *Planning* a new task requires children to formulate a concept or idea of what needs to be done. *Organizing* the information requires them to coordinate pertinent information from all of the senses to formulate a plan, sequence, and time the movement. This phase requires children to have a good sense of self. They must know subconsciously how their bodies are put together and how they physically relate to things in their environment. The brain must also know how to move to accomplish the task. This is learned through the process of trial and error as the child develops and then practices a skill. The successes and corrective measures learned in movement are the result of feedback and memory of those lessons. The products of the feedback process are body scheme, memory of motor movements, and skilled, well-coordinated movements. *Sequencing* the steps of the task and being able to perform body movements at the correct time and in the correct order also requires feedforward motor control. The child is required to project what he or she needs to do into the future (feedforward). For example, when kicking a rolling ball, children must know exactly when and where that ball will meet their body. They must plan where to

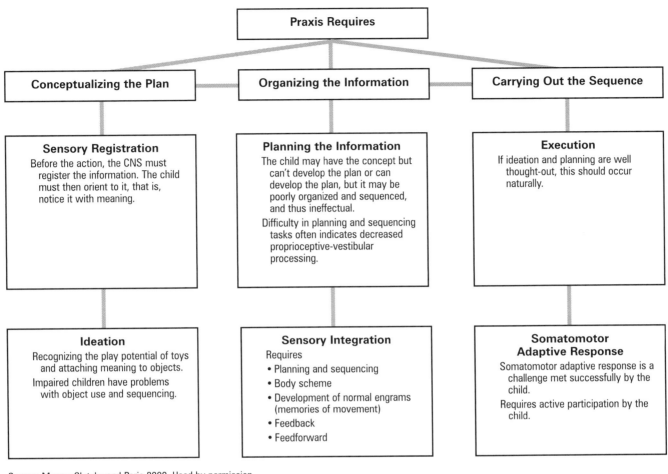

Praxis Requires		
Conceptualizing the Plan	**Organizing the Information**	**Carrying Out the Sequence**
Sensory Registration Before the action, the CNS must register the information. The child must then orient to it, that is, notice it with meaning.	**Planning the Information** The child may have the concept but can't develop the plan or can develop the plan, but it may be poorly organized and sequenced, and thus ineffectual. Difficulty in planning and sequencing tasks often indicates decreased proprioceptive-vestibular processing.	**Execution** If ideation and planning are well thought-out, this should occur naturally.
Ideation Recognizing the play potential of toys and attaching meaning to objects. Impaired children have problems with object use and sequencing.	**Sensory Integration** Requires • Planning and sequencing • Body scheme • Development of normal engrams (memories of movement) • Feedback • Feedforward	**Somatomotor Adaptive Response** Somatomotor adaptive response is a challenge met successfully by the child. Requires active participation by the child.

Source: Murray-Slutsky and Paris 2000. Used by permission.

Figure 2.3   Requirements of praxis

move their bodies to kick the ball and prepare to kick the ball at the exact moment the ball is in front of their feet. This process requires timing and sequencing of the motor movements of both the leg and trunk. Feedback occurs after the task is executed and children learn from their successes and failures. *Execution* of smooth coordinated movements and functional activities occurs naturally if the child has planned and organized the information effectively.

Motor planning is the process required to learn a skill. Motor planning occurs only while the child is learning new tasks, performing unfamiliar tasks, or adapting a previously learned skill. It requires that the child actively participate, figuring out what to do and how to do it. Changing the activity or the environment in which the activity is performed requires changes in the motor plan. However, once the child has learned the activity and performs it automatically and proficiently in all environments, it no longer requires motor planning.

Motor planning is the conscious attention and effort required to master a new activity. When children are learning to motor plan a new task, such as tying their shoes, they must pay attention to their fingers and the shoelaces and organize and sequence the task into its component steps. Once children are able to complete the task several times, they no longer need to concentrate on it. Their fingers automatically receive the motor plan, and tying their shoes becomes a skill that can be accomplished in any environment (Murray-Slutsky and Paris 2000).

Any task that requires learning and attention will require motor planning until it can be accomplished without conscious attention. Motor planning is required to put on clothes, eat, speak, write, play with toys, use tools, and participate in new games or any sport. Once children learn the activity, the brain automatically tells their muscles what to do.

Dyspraxia or Practic Dysfunction

Dyspraxia is a motor planning problem in which children have difficulty planning, organizing, or carrying out a sequence of unfamiliar actions. Dyspraxic children will require more repetition to learn new tasks or activities and, once learned, they will have difficulty transferring their knowledge to new situations. Self-care activities, such as dressing, bathing, and eating, will be difficult until they have been mastered in multiple environments. Sports and extracurricular activities like bicycling or skating will be difficult for these children as they focus on perfecting the timing and sequencing of new motor movements. Children may have articulation difficulties or difficulty sequencing words or letters. Handwriting will be hard because of the ever-changing sequence of letters and motor movements. Taking information from their mind, then organizing and sequencing it into a motor act is very difficult; however, the task becomes even harder when the child has to write creatively from memory. Planning and sequencing words to tell a story is hard enough, but to put it on paper requires even more complex motor planning.

Gubbay (1975) believed that in using standardized psychological testing, the single most important criterion for diagnosing dyspraxia is a significantly lower performance IQ compared to a verbal IQ. Significantly lower is described as at least a 15-point discrepancy. Gubbay's theory identifies dyspraxia as a dysfunction in which the child cognitively knows what is expected but is motorically unable to produce the desired response. This is an accurate definition of dyspraxia for testable children without speech and language difficulties; however, a child may have dyspraxia even if he or she does not show a discrepancy between verbal and performance measures.

Children with dyspraxia may learn to use compensatory strategies in an attempt to be successful. They may rely on cognitive strategies, such as memorizing each step of a task, whereas their peers tend to have an innate ability to perform the tasks. These cognitive strategies are exhausting to these children because they make them work much harder than their peers and don't always work. Memorization of tasks is a strategy that works only in the environments and under the conditions in which the tasks were learned. The child will have difficulty modifying the task under new conditions, performing it in different environments, or adding to the task to make it part of a more complex sequence.

Motor incoordination, motor clumsiness, and awkwardness are frequently seen in children with dyspraxia because of the combination of inefficient processing of sensory information and their difficulty organizing, planning, and sequencing motor movements. Motor control issues are secondary to sensory processing problems. The body scheme is poorly established and the motor movements appear disorganized. The problem is on a subcortical level and involves the brain's ability to receive, organize, and process sensory information. In typical development, as the child moves, the movement helps integrate the sensory information and develop body scheme. However, according to Ayres (1972), "if the information which the body perceives from its somatosensory receptors is not precise, the brain has a poor basis from which to build its body scheme of the body" (p. 170).

Sensory Integrative-Based Dyspraxia

Bundy, Lane, and Murray (2002) describe sensory integrative-based dyspraxia as deficits in processing one or more types of sensation. Different types of dyspraxia are associated with dysfunctions in different sensory systems. Overlap occurs within the sensory systems so increasingly more complex dysfunctions may occur. The authors describe the relationship between dyspraxia and the sensory systems as follows:

- *Postural deficits* in extensor muscle tone, prone extension, proximal stability, supine flexion, and/or equilibrium reactions can result from dysfunctions in processing visual, vestibular, or proprioceptive input. These may further lead to the practic dysfunction:

  - *Bilateral integration and sequencings.* This is a motor planning problem that affects the child's coordination and sequencing. It is a sensory-based problem that is hypothesized to originate within the vestibular and proprioceptive systems. Children have difficulty using the two sides of their body together in a coordinated fashion. They often fail to develop a skilled hand dominance or preference, avoid crossing the midline of their body, and experience difficulty with anticipating movements or projected action sequences (feedforward). Difficulty with bilateral motor control (using the two sides of the body together) may affect hopping, skipping, jumping, doing jumping jacks, and symmetrical and reciprocal stride jumping.

- *Discrimination disorders* result from dysfunctions in processing visual, vestibular, proprioceptive, tactile, or auditory input. Tactile discrimination disorder is the most common disorder and involves underresponsiveness to tactile and proprioceptive sensory input. The child has difficulty discriminating touch and information from his joints. The child may have any combination of fine motor, gross motor, and oral-motor problems. Discrimination disorders may lead to:

  - *Somatodyspraxia.* This is a motor planning problem that is hypothesized to originate from difficulties within the tactile and proprioceptive systems but also includes vestibular and often auditory difficulties. Children appear clumsy; have poor tactile discrimination and body scheme; fine motor, gross motor, and oral-motor problems; problems in construction or manipulative play; difficulties with feedback and feedforward (projected action sequences); and praxis-related skills.

Behavioral and Emotional Characteristics of Dyspraxia

Children have an innate drive to be successful and to feel competent. The moment children have to interact purposefully with their environment, motor planning is required. It doesn't take long for children to realize that once they have mastered a task, they can successfully accomplish it only if it is performed in the same environment. Therefore, to be successful and to avoid stress, children quickly learn the need for control.

They must control everything: what clothes are worn, which activities are performed, and how they are completed. They will need to control what, where, and when they eat. Because transitions and change involve motor planning a new activity, which often is accompanied by anxiety and stress, these children must control where they go. The more they can control, the more they can assure that they will be able to function. Often, dyspraxia can be identified just by the parents' description of the child's need to be controlling from birth. As children improve in body scheme and motor planning skills, new activities can be introduced; and as they learn that they possess the skills to be successful and gain body awareness and self-esteem, their need for control will gradually disappear.

If children have strong language skills, as in a child with Asperger's syndrome, they actually may show a higher verbal IQ than a performance IQ. They may prefer to talk about what needs to be done, rather than actually doing it. They may be able to describe the beautiful picture that they are drawing, while the actual strokes on the paper are unrecognizable. Other children may frantically beg to do every activity, but then may be unable to sustain attention or organize themselves to complete any task. They may run from activity to activity saying, "I know what I want to do. It's this...No it's this...No it's this." When asked what they want to do, dyspraxic children cannot tell their plan. Often their response is, "I'll show you."

These children are unable to organize themselves, much less their belongings, desks, or papers. Their clothing may be disheveled: shirts untucked and shoes untied—tasks that require motor planning and body awareness. They forget their books, lunch boxes, papers, and assignments. Their apparent lack of sense of time, coupled with their disorganization, results in their being constantly late and not turning in assignments or finishing projects. They appear distractible, inattentive, hyperactive, or disorganized as a secondary characteristic of dyspraxia.

These children are aware of how much harder they have to work than their peers. Everything they do is a struggle that requires tremendous effort and concentration. Their emotional state is fragile and their self-confidence tentative. They realize how others react to them, and they recognize that they are awkward and clumsy. These observations, coupled with their poor sense of self, often results in feelings of insecurity and a loss of inner drive to successfully encounter the world. They may demonstrate emotional instability. They may be unable to deal with small roadblocks, such as broken lead in a pencil, and will fall apart, crying hysterically. Some may act babylike and immature or be unable to separate from their parents. If these children encounter any difficulty or failure, they may never try again. If they muster up the energy to attempt a task, their efforts must be rewarded by success (Murray-Slutsky and Paris 2000).

Evaluating a Child With Sensory Integrative Problems

Children's behaviors give us concrete clues about their sensory processing. Their likes, dislikes, persistence (or lack of it) at a task, emotional responses, motor coordination, and language are all integral parts in assessing their processing. Their behaviors, or output, serve to objectify what we cannot see occurring within the nervous system (sensory processing).

Through tracking children's behaviors we can obtain a clear view of how they respond to sensory information. This requires meticulously listing children's behaviors, desires or obtaining behaviors, and dislikes or avoidance behaviors and correlating these behaviors with the appropriate sensory system. This information can be used to determine how children process sensory stimulus or discriminate sensory information.

Observing the child's behavior and behavior checklists or questionnaires are methods of obtaining needed sensory information. For example, the *Sensory Profile* (Dunn 1999) is a standard method for professionals to measure a child's sensory processing abilities and to profile the effects of sensory processing on functional performance in the daily life of the child. It is a judgment-based caregiver questionnaire. This questionnaire describes typical functional problems and behaviors that are caused by sensory processing problems. It provides professionals a picture of the child's strengths, concerns, and performance during daily life. The child's overall performance and responses, or lack of responses, to auditory, visual, vestibular, tactile, and multisensory processing is summarized and compared to that of other children. For the professional who is trained in sensory integrative theory and practice, it provides a basis from which to conduct further testing and to hypothesize about the child's sensory processing.

Objective testing of skills and performance is needed to analyze the impact sensory stimulus difficulties have on the child's ability to function. Central processing of the sensory input, the ability to organize sensory information for use, is needed to achieve adaptive responses and functional performances. By tracking the child's behavioral, emotional, and sensory responses with his physical performance, a therapist trained in sensory integration identifies patterns that have clinical significance. Discrimination disorders, dyspraxia, or modulation disorders (central processing difficulties) are complex dysfunctions that can be determined through testing but require an expert knowledgeable in sensory processing.

Children who fit the picture of having a sensory integrative disorder should receive an evaluation by a qualified occupational or physical therapist who has received postgraduate training in sensory integrative theory and treatment or who has pursued certification or continuing education in this area. Results of the evaluation will indicate whether the child has SI dysfunction and provide a profile of the child's sensory processing abilities in a number of areas.

Evaluations consist of both standardized testing and structured observations of responses to sensory stimulation, posture, balance, coordination, and eye movements. The occupational or physical therapist conducting the testing may also observe spontaneous play.

The purpose of testing lies in determining the underlying problem in order to establish and implement an effective intervention program designed to remediate it. Intervention frequently entails sensory integrative treatment programs designed and implemented by a therapist skilled in sensory integration, as well as sensory diets (see chapter 10).

For more detailed information about sensory integration and disorders of sensory integration, refer to *Exploring the Spectrum of Autism and Pervasive Developmental Disorders: Intervention Strategies* by Murray-Slutsky and Paris (2000) or visit www.starservices.tv, www.sinetwork.org, or www.SPDnetwork.org.

Deviations in Development: The Impact on Behavior

3

How Learning Occurs in Development

As therapists we are constantly involved with evaluating children and their development. We look not only for developmental milestones, but also at how a child interacts, moves, communicates, and problem-solves. We also look for developing skills that will lead to higher-level abilities to meet life's challenges. We have recognized that children who experience deviations in their development use behaviors to cope with the challenges and to communicate with others. It is often the coping strategy a child uses that clues us to look further at sensory processing, skill development, and a child's self-esteem to determine where he may need help or intervention and avoid the need for problematic coping strategies (behavior). While all children exhibit worrisome behaviors at one time or another, there are elements in development that, when problems occur and these elements are missed, will certainly result in problematic behaviors that may be the expression of not only a coping strategy but also a more deeply rooted medical or developmental issue. Our intent is to review some important elements of development and how they relate to behavior.

All children have a need to function within their environment, and behaviors arise out of that need. Children with impaired development need to function just as typical children do, but are hindered by more challenges than their typically developing peers. Because they encounter more challenges in the course of their efforts to perform, they are more prone to difficult behaviors as they try to cope. Once the behaviors are learned, children then believe that it is normal to use the behaviors to cope with their difficulties and will repeat the behaviors, believing them to be acceptable and the only way to deal with difficulty. Addressing the behaviors involves using behavioral strategies to teach alternative coping methods and behaviors, and addressing the underlying developmental difficulty.

Infants

Babies, toddlers, and young children typically learn through imitation, movement, and play. Early play experiences usually begin around three months of age with infants mimicking faces and sounds. These reciprocal interactions are a keystone to developing social interactions and the imitation skills needed for future learning, communication, and higher-order skills. Their absence may be an indicator of such conditions as genetic disorders or sensory processing difficulties (visual impairments, deafness, sensory modulation, autism-spectrum disorders, and others).

As they develop the ability to move, children increase their strength, self-organization and coordination through repeating new movements in increasingly challenging ways. Total-body play experiences enhance the ability to organize sensations for use in creating more complex environmental interactions and adaptive behaviors. Children who are unable to tolerate positions or move in normal patterns, skip or alter other areas of development, such as:

- development of the strength in muscle groups needed for motor control (gross or fine motor skills and language),

- development of knowledge of their body and of their environment,

- coordination,

- learning to organize or regulate themselves, and

- visual-motor skills.

For example, children who avoid crawling due to a sensory processing problem avoid the precise activity needed to develop their arm and hand muscles for feeding, writing, and other fine motor skills. Their environmental interactions and adaptive behaviors may become very restrictive, in that they will avoid what they find uncomfortable or intolerable. These same children may later refuse paper and pencil tasks because they lack the development needed to hold and control those items.

Babies with a neurological condition or torticollis (wry neck), who roll in only one direction, may develop a neglect of the opposite side of their body, lack certain hand functions, and have restrictions in their visual field that are important to function. By six months of age many will avoid uncomfortable positions, avoid weight-bearing needed for development, and have diminished hand use.

Children who do not develop postural control or who cannot tolerate certain sensory experiences may become controlling and inflexible in their routines and in dealings with others. They may avoid the need to use postural control and avoid sensory experiences.

Carlton, as an infant, displayed low tone and did not crawl; as a 4-year-old with postural control problems, he would not go onto the playground with his class. Try as they might, the staff could not get Carlton to leave the fenced gateway to play with his classmates unless a staff member held his hand and walked him into the sandy play area. If left alone at this point, he would drop to the ground and refuse to move unless someone came to his aid. Carlton also insisted on help to walk to the cafeteria. It involved leaving his portable classroom, walking down steps or a ramp, and walking across grass to get to a sidewalk. If the staff refused him, he would drop to the ground and refuse to walk. Staff members thought him difficult and controlling, when the problem stemmed from poor postural control and ability to control his body.

Later, children typically begin imitating those with whom they come in contact. Facial expressions, vocal play and intonation, speech patterns, and motor sequences are all learned through imitation. Children with sensory processing difficulties and disorders like autism-spectrum disorders may not register or notice another person or may not engage in imitation and fail to develop these pre-language and social-interaction skills.

Toddlers

At about age one, children will progress from playing with toys in a cause-effect manner and begin learning how use of their body and extremities can have a direct impact on their environment. As typically developing children become more organized in their ability to perform, learn to manipulate objects, move through their environment, and interact with people and things in that environment, cause and effect combined with feedback from their interactions allow them to develop an internal map of their body (body scheme). Concepts of directionality, spatial relationships (e.g., near-far; big-small; up-down and in-out), and complex motor skills are based upon a good body scheme.

The child who is disorganized due to sensory processing problems or hampered by syndromes, neurological conditions, or other medical issues may not move in normal patterns of movement, and may develop use of bizarre motor patterns, avoidance behaviors, and tantrums. There are two sequelae to this. In the low-functioning case, these children may not only fail to develop a good body scheme, but also fail to develop cause and effect. Cause and effect is learned through feedback. When children cannot learn from their own feedback, there is a severe impediment to learning. Early cause and effect is the underlying concept to many higher-level skills. In the case of impaired body scheme in the presence of cause and effect, coordination may be impaired, affecting the ability to perform complex motor skills, such as jumping jacks, hopscotch, or sports-related movements. These children may be very clumsy, fall often, and not be able to keep up with other children in play. Their perception of spatial relationships and abstract concepts of time and movement through space can be negatively affected and lead to problems in developing higher-order cognitive skills: learning to write or perform complex math skills and analytical thinking.

The young toddler begins to use symbolic play to replicate real life: taking care of a baby doll, cooking, or housekeeping. Symbolic or imaginary play allows young children to relate objects to their bodies, such as using a comb or hairbrush; placing objects into containers, sorting by similarities, imitating role models, and eventually establishing their own personas and interests. They begin to relate to others with shared interests and discoveries and, by the age of four, begin to play cooperatively with other children. As imaginary play develops, they will create new opportunities for problem solving and new challenges.

Night terrors and the fear of sleeping alone often are behaviors that crop up in toddlers. It is important to remember that toddlers often cannot discern imaginary experiences from reality. Things seen in the movies or television and dreams are all very real at this stage of typical development. These often are the cause of disrupted sleep patterns, the inability of the toddler to calm himself and to fall back to sleep, and the fear of separation from parents. They can also lead to avoidance of going to bed and sleeping alone, night terrors, and anxieties in the young child.

Children learn to label objects and expand their language skills through play. Toddlers learn to question, learn social skill interactions, and begin to use descriptive language. Receptive and expressive language develops through these experiences. Children of this age begin to identify their wants and needs and the people in their environment, and they feel empowered by language. Tantrums (common to toddlers) are a strategy used before communication evolves or is sufficient to convey what the toddler wants to express. As language increases and negotiation becomes an art, they offer the toddler alternatives to the use of tantrums for communication.

School-Age Children

In school-age children, play sequences are expanded, step-by-step, becoming longer and more complex. Sharing and cooperation continue to develop. Through play, children learn role delineation and social interaction; recognize, label, and learn to cope with their emotions; and learn rules about the boundaries of acceptable behavior. They build their self-esteem through mastery of ever-increasing complexities of function. They carve out a place in society with these skills and are able to develop relationships with peers and function within the context of their daily lives.

At school, learning is sequential, and knowledge is scaffolded upon material and skills learned in earlier grades. Motor skills typically developed in the earlier stages of development combine with visual and auditory skills, contribute to attention, and allow the formation of more complex tasks involving writing, complex mathematical equations, and larger vocabularies. Children with gaps in their development may have impediments to learning. They rapidly grow frustrated with the fight to keep up with their peers. Behaviors can emerge unexpectedly, be misinterpreted for willful misbehavior or disobedience, and not be recognized as a symptom of a more deeply rooted problem.

Motor control, for some children, can be a fluctuating commodity. As children gain the core stability and extremity motor control needed to master the challenges they face, competency and self-esteem increase. However, for some children, postural or core stability is lost during *growth spurts,* leaving them to struggle once again to gain previous levels of competency with their new body size. The simplest tasks become seemingly insurmountable, frustrating the child and sapping him of his self-esteem. Children struggling to maintain self-regulation (attention and focus) may regress during growth spurts as they lose their core stability. As functional skills regress, behaviors can emerge.

Any roadblock in normal development can create an opportunity in which behavioral difficulties can surface. Behavioral difficulties can occur as children try to compensate for or avoid their weakness, struggling to develop coping strategies that work for them. In these cases, the behaviors are caused by a lag in a specific area of development or a skill that is missing. While we know the cause for the behavioral problems, we cannot excuse behaviors that are maladaptive. Programs that address both the missing skills and the troublesome behavioral coping strategy have proven to be the most effective. Our goal is to have a happy, well-adjusted child who has the skills to use appropriate and acceptable coping strategies.

Behavioral Problems Seen in Infants, Toddlers, and Older Children

Social Interaction

Social interaction and communication skills are of paramount importance to learning. The noted psychologist, Vygotsky, felt that social interaction is the key to cognitive growth (1978). A child learns through interactions and experiences shared with others—parents, teachers, siblings, and friends.

Difficulty relating to or interacting with others and making friends is often seen in children with sensory processing disorders (sensory integrative difficulties), learning disabilities, attention deficit disorders, developmental delays, and in children on the autism spectrum. This may present in the infant as a failure to bond well with parents; a failure to engage in facial and vocal play; and perhaps even an aversion to being held, cuddled, or rocked by family members. Young children may not engage their peers and often do not make eye contact unless taught and then prompted to do so. They may appear absent from or indifferent to the goings-on around them. In either of these instances the child may focus instead on parts of a toy or the lights in the room, look through a window, fall asleep, or hide, rather than engaging in or observing what may be happening in the room. Some have been erroneously suspected of being deaf for this very reason. Imaginative play may be absent or impaired. If it is taught, it may occur within a restricted context or robotically. The child will not spontaneously vary his play. Some children may be so restricted in their ability to play that they simply mouth objects or throw them.

Other infants may be totally overwhelmed by their environment and lack of understanding as to what is happening or expected. Sensory problems often play a major role in these children, causing them to be easily agitated and disgruntled, difficult to calm, and unable to separate from their parent or caretaker to engage and learn.

Successful interaction with others requires children to be aware of their environment and to develop basic play and social skills that allow for a gradual increase in complex interaction with others. Older children who fail to develop play and social skills will have trouble relating to others. Their behaviors will range from playing in parallel but not cooperatively with other children, insistence on playing only one game, refusals at turn-taking, or aggressive reactions toward others. They may develop behaviors that keep others at a distance. Some poke at others with their fingers, some use sticks, and others lash out by hitting, kicking, or biting, making the behavior a high priority for change. They may appear very egocentric and not interested in what other children want. They typically do not greet people they meet and cannot engage in pretend play. They may function in a very literal sense: unable to engage their peers in shared interests or sustain a conversation. They may avoid eye contact. They have difficulty making and keeping friends, have trouble sharing interests of others, choosing instead to focus only on what interests them. They may become the subject of ridicule, be teased, or be ostracized by their peers. Behavioral problems may ensue as the child tries to overcome a low self-esteem and reacts to peers using less than optimal problem solving and social skills.

Some children miss or do not understand the unspoken rules of social interactions by observing how others respond in different situations, as do typical children. The implied meaning of a frown or grimace may simply be lost on these children. They may not register the disapproval in an adult's voice. When children fail to read situations and do not alter their behavior appropriately for the given situation, they must be taught in very concrete terms what are acceptable behaviors and what are not. These strategies are clearly delineated in chapter 8, Behavioral Intervention Techniques.

Communication

Functional speech eludes many children with atypical or delayed development, making it difficult or impossible for them to express their emotions or reactions, make simple requests, answer simple questions, or ask the millions of questions a typical child would pose. Speech and communication problems set these children up for behavioral difficulties in social interactions as they attempt to communicate their needs and wants. They are often unable to ask why something is occurring, and may not understand what is expected. The strategies they use are their "best attempt" to communicate and cope. When these strategies are ineffective or result in difficult behaviors, it is our responsibility to help them learn effective replacement behaviors (coping strategies), while we improve their communication skills.

Nonverbal Communication and Behavior

Many children with pervasive developmental delays, autism spectrum, other developmental disorders, and genetic disorders have communication disorders apart from speech issues. Children may also lack the ability to spontaneously initiate, use, and sustain *nonverbal* forms of communication. They may not initiate pointing, gesture, or mime to make themselves understood in the absence of verbal communication. They may have deficits in the ability to use sustained eye contact, facial expressions, or body language. This hinders their ability to communicate in social interactions, but also limits their ability to learn. Learning is based not only on independent exploration and experience, but on reciprocal interactions between the child and another person. In the absence of verbal communication, nonverbal skills must be relied upon and are an important component of communication and a key to comprehension or understanding.

When children have no acceptable way to communicate and are not taught or prompted to use an acceptable method of communication, they will find a way to get their needs met—often utilizing behaviors that are challenging. Their atypical and unconventional methods of communication may include throwing themselves on the floor; throwing objects that they have no interest in; ripping paper or books; pulling at others' jewelry, hair, or clothing; and hitting. They may fail to be accepted or understood, may learn or interpret new information incorrectly, or even be removed from school or play because of their behavior.

Expressive Language Problems

Young children, at about two-and-a-half to three years old, will go through a phase of asking the same questions over and over again: "Why?" or "What's this?" are common. However, in children with pervasive developmental delay, autism, Asperger's, or sensory processing disorders who are able to question, behaviors often include a litany of ritualized, one-sided questions with a lack of interest in the answers. They often change topics rapidly, not noticing that the other person is not following what is said and perhaps has lost interest. They may not notice and often will not respond to questions posed to them during conversation, or they will answer the question in the same way each time it is posed. In those children with speech, it may be robotic in its tone and rhythm. These children may mimic melodies but not enunciate words correctly. They may exhibit an echolalia, either repeating what is said to them or what they hear from others or on the television. Parents may be fooled into believing that their child understands, because he talks, but echolalia is not the same as understanding what is being said. Labeling of objects may be impaired, and information gained from descriptive language may be faulty or even meaningless. Other children may develop complex speech, with errors that appear odd or peculiar; for example, their language may be devoid of descriptives.

Receptive Language Problems: Comprehension

Another dependent variable of learning is comprehension, whether of verbal or nonverbal means. If children lack comprehension, they cannot learn easily and reliably. A child with language impairments may not comprehend what the adult perceives is the pertinent component of the experience but may form an entirely unpredicted and erroneous conclusion or rule (Murray-Slutsky and Paris 2000). It is critical that the child perceive the important component that you are trying to teach. Imagine trying to teach a child the letter *A* , and the child only focuses on the color red that it is written in. Every time you show the child the letter *A* , he focuses on and responds with "red." Visual cues and communication strategies are often helpful in conveying information to the child with receptive language problems. It is important that we assure the child is processing and focusing on the part of the message we are trying to teach.

In several disorders, Asperger's syndrome being one, children use a vocabulary that is far advanced for their age, sounding like little professors. Because of the words the children use, adults presume a level of comprehension that they do not have. Comprehension may well be lower than their word use would suggest. In these cases, as well as with children with auditory processing impairments, fluid in their ears, or receptive language impairment, the child may misunderstand what is said or be unable to discriminate between words. His behavior may be taken for disobedience rather than poor comprehension.

Children with Asperger's syndrome, autism, or pervasive developmental disorder have disparities in their capabilities. These children may learn to read at a very early age, before the age of three, or may perform complex math skills well in advance of their age level. Grammatical structure of sentences may be immature, speech limited to repetitive phrases, topics, or repetition of scripts from a favorite video, DVD, or cartoon, and may not be contiguous with the topic of discussion. These children may not be able to follow simple instructions or remember to bring homework home. The discrepancy between the child's perceived advanced intellectual abilities and his difficulties functioning may result in his being labeled as defiant or lazy.

Children with speech and communication problems have never experienced normal communication. When children are unable to understand what is expected or to communicate what they want, behaviors (particularly tantrums) may develop as a method of requesting and then clarifying requests. Tantrums can easily be reinforced and become a learned behavior if not dealt with appropriately. See chapter 9, Handling Temper Tantrums and Challenging Behaviors, for more information on tantrums.

Children with communication difficulties may exhibit an emotional response that may be inappropriate for the situation or not match the message they are trying to communicate. For example, they may laugh or smile when telling you someone is hurt. Their inappropriate responses and emotional reactions may appear defiant or insulting, provoking feelings of anger in the adult dealing with their behavior. We cannot be certain that they comprehend the information the way it was intended and that they understand the implied meaning of a situation. They may voice an inappropriate reaction, their facial expressions may not match the message they are delivering, they may cry or behave oddly, not follow simple commands, or appear simply not to listen to instructions. They are labeled as being poorly behaved when they honestly do not understand what is being said to them. What appears to be a willful defiant response may actually be a learned behavior, based on poor comprehension and processing.

Stereotypic, Restricted Behaviors, Interest, or Activity

Children with autism, fragile X, Soto's, and other syndromes demonstrate repetitive behaviors and activities. They may flap their hands, exhibit whole-body rocking, hold their hands in front of their eyes, or become aggressive toward themselves or others, to name just a few behaviors. Children with sensory processing disorders, learning disabilities, and attention-deficit disorder have shown restricted behaviors, interests, and activities as well as obsessive tendencies. Parents grow frustrated attempting to extinguish these behaviors, not knowing that many stem from the types of sensory processing difficulties described in chapter 2. For more information on identifying the sensory basis of stereotypic behaviors and intervention strategies, refer to appendix C.

To complicate matters, although most children learn by building ever more complex sequences of behavior in order to function, there are those who do not. They are Gestalt learners, who take in the total experience when learning a new task or information. This may include the setting, the exact words used by the instructor, the exact piece of equipment used, the lighting, the background sounds, and often a myriad of extraneous information. For most, this method of learning is not a problem. However, some Gestalt learners learn by memorization, and may function only in rote memory. Those with conditions such as autism and pervasive developmental delay may not extract the pertinent from the nonpertinent information or may not be able to break down the information into subsets that can be used in other tasks. In either case they are not easily able to generalize the information between settings, with new equipment, or with new people. Learning tends to be all or none, and very situation-specific, making it very restricted. Children with autism-spectrum and pervasive developmental delay do not often recognize the steps in the process and cannot break a task down when they need to alter it. By not being able to break a task down, they are not easily able to use a step-by-step process to build the more complex sequences that typical children do. These children may be the ones who learn to sight-read whole words rather than learning to spell by each letter to build words, and they prefer numbers (math), factual information, and historical data to the ever-changing demands of writing, spelling, and other school-related tasks. They may exhibit problems in praxis. For more information on praxis, see chapter 2.

Overfocusing on parts of objects is a coping behavior. Lovaas et al. (1971) proposed that children with autism may fail to manage multiple stimuli within their environment. This is also true of children with sensory processing disorders. When these children are presented with multiple stimuli, they tend to overfocus on one mode of sensory input rather than integrating all of the presenting stimuli (Murray-Slutsky and Paris 2000). The child who spins the wheels of a toy car instead of playing appropriately with it may be overfocusing to the exclusion of all other sensory inputs. School-age children may display intense fascinations or obsessions with machines such as computers, video games, or televisions. They may also block out learning in school by playing or fidgeting with their pencils or other objects at their desks. These behaviors often interfere with learning and become a high priority for change. While improving the child's ability to process multisensory information would be the primary goal that would address the core problem, altering the child's behavior to enhance learning becomes a simultaneous goal.

Perseveration Behavior

Children who are hindered in their attempts to play are hindered in their ability to learn. The child who cannot initiate play and sustain it; who cannot interact spontaneously with adults or peers to share interests; or who is unable to imitate is severely hampered in learning. Some are hampered by a neurological process called perseveration: repetitious motor acts or vocalizations and an inability to stop or change the behavior. This is not a willful behavior, nor is it a ritualistic behavior. Their play is restricted only to actions they have learned, repeating them over and over. Their inflexibility and lack of creativity do not allow them to master new challenges in their environment, learn new information, or expand their capabilities.

Rituals and Routines

Children with developmental disorders, sensory processing disorders, and autism-spectrum disorders tend to formulate rules about how the world works and about what they learn. Because of faulty sensory processing, rules may be learned incompletely, out of context, and with distortions.

Children with impaired receptive communication and difficulty with understanding what is happening may have difficulty transitioning between activities. Once engaged, they are unwilling to terminate the activity to move on to another. The interruption is viewed as a violation or intrusion that will trigger a tantrum, screams of frustration, distress, and/or avoidance behaviors. Rituals become the child's way of coping. Rituals are developed to engineer the environment, the task demand, and even the conversation so that the child can cope. Strict adherence to rituals lets the child predict what will happen next and allows him to function. These children learn best in highly structured settings, devoid of extraneous tasks and visual and auditory stimulation that will complicate learning. Environmental modifications, identified in chapter 7, often enhance the child's learning and diminish residual behavioral difficulties. Concrete behavioral strategies, identified in chapter 8, are useful in objectifying teaching.

Neurologically Based Behaviors

Neurological differences in autism and other disorders have been associated with the learning and behavior difficulties that accompany some developmental disorders. The neurological differences have been associated with disregulated emotional tone and impaired processing of memory needed for learning and motivation. Specific behaviors stemming from these alterations have included:

- purposeless hyperactivity
- impaired social interaction
- stereotyped motor behavior
- disordered responses to novel or new stimuli
- a lack of recognition of objects and situations
- poor visual and tactile memory for learning
- impaired learning processes
- impaired auditory sense:
    - lack of recognition of specific tones and intensities
    - poor localization of sound

- poor ability to distinguish between like-sounding words (e.g., fish and dish; dog and log; fight and fly)

- impaired auditory memory and inability to follow multiple-step instructions

Biochemical and seizure activity have also been discussed in the literature as being the cause of stereotypic, repetitive, and self-injurious behaviors.

Summary

Developmentally based issues are often at the roots of behavioral chaos and must be considered when analyzing and prioritizing problems to be addressed. Behaviors may be seen in any combination and in the presence of a variety of disorders, including sensory processing disorders, learning disabilities, attention-deficit disorder, developmental disorders, autism and Asperger's syndrome, and others. They also are seen in children who have no medical diagnoses. Sometimes behavior problems are the first indication that a child may have a sensory processing disorder, a developmental delay, or a skill not developed. Although the behaviors may be frustrating, it is important to recognize that they are not willful, and not always sensory in nature. There are multiple causes for behaviors, namely communicative disorders, problems in motor control development, and sensory processing disorders.

Although behavioral challenges are chaotic and daunting, children with atypical development or other disorders can and do learn, and are capable of learning new behaviors and coping strategies. In most children who have a sensory-related behavior problem, the problem will be both sensory and behavioral. The underlying sensory issues must be addressed through treatment if we hope to alter behaviors. In addition to treating the underlying sensory problem, these children must specifically be taught behaviors that are appropriate and acceptable. We must help them develop the skills needed to cope with life's demands; teach the social skills needed for successful interactions; and identify strategies that will aid them in regulating their emotional tone and coping with the stress of ever-changing situations and schedules, to organize them for function. The methodology outlined in this book, in the tables, and in the worksheets, incorporates developmental difficulties as a cause of problematic behavior and outline strategies to use in addressing the underlying problems.

Basic Concepts: Analyzing Behaviors

4

How do we start to identify the order that exists within chaos? A child's behavior may mean one thing in one environment and something else in another. Two different children may do the same behavior for totally different reasons. Children are complicated and nonlinear; they do things for multiple reasons. How do we identify them and prioritize them to come up with a comprehensive plan?

To unravel the chaos we need to look systematically at the behaviors and the environments in which they occur. This system, while presented in a linear, step-by-step fashion, is truly nonlinear. The causes for each behavior must be analyzed continually, taking into consideration environmental factors that either help or hinder the child from gaining control over his behaviors. Children's neurological systems and how intensely they register sensory information (hypo- or hypersensitive), their arousal level at the time the behavior occurred, and their ability to self-regulate are all major factors in solving the mystery. Identifying whether changing the behavior is a priority is just one of the items that must be adjusted based on sensory and environmental factors. A plan often addresses multiple issues rather than just one behavior. Children require a nonlinear strategy to help them function better within their environment as well as behave appropriately.

Children Behave for Reasons: Primary Cause

There is always a reason why children do what they do. Simply put, they are either trying to *obtain* something or *avoid* it. O'Neil et al. (1990) looked at the functional assessment of problematic behaviors. They believed that all behaviors served the function to get/obtain (attention, self-stimulation, item, or activity) or to escape/avoid (demand/request, item or activity, or person). Durand (1990) believed difficult behaviors arise from the need for attention, to escape, to obtain something tangible, or for sensory reasons. O'Neil et al. and Durand both identified sensory as a function served by behaviors; however, they discussed sensory primarily in terms of sensory stimulation behaviors or severe self-abusive behaviors. Neither addressed the role sensory integrative or sensory processing difficulties have on the function of behaviors.

In our book, *Exploring the Spectrum of Autism and Pervasive Developmental Disorders: Intervention Strategies,* we addressed the function of behaviors taking into account both behavioral and sensory integrative reasons (Murray-Slutsky and Paris 2000). We agree that behaviors serve two functions: to obtain or to avoid something. However, we believe that the child is trying to either obtain or avoid for the purpose of communication (to obtain or avoid attention or a task, object, or activity) or for internal/systemic (sensory) reasons. Internal/systemic is further divided into visceral needs that are from the child's internal sensory environment (pain, hunger, or autoimmune responses) or sensory needs, which address the child's sensory threshold as either over- or under-responsive.

Sensory behaviors are either sensory-obtaining (underresponsive) or avoiding (over-responsive). Nonproductive self-stimulatory sensory behaviors (identified as sensory-obtaining behaviors), are differentiated from productive sensory behaviors that are used in an attempt to calm and organize.

We identify behaviors resulting from dyspraxia, motor-planning, and motor control difficulties. They are addressed both as sensory-based behaviors and specifically under task avoidance (communication). In order to tease out the specific underlying cause for the behaviors, the following analysis must be completed:

- Task analysis (What does the task require?),

- Skills analysis (Does the child possess the needed skills for the task?), and

- Emotional analysis (What is the child's emotional reaction to the activity?) (Murray-Slutsky and Paris 2000).

Behaviors are provoked by situations and events in the child's life. How the child responds to these events (i.e., his behaviors) is governed by the child's sensory and behavioral needs. These behaviors stem either from the need to obtain something the child wants or to avoid something the child does not want. Problematic and challenging behaviors first develop to meet one of these needs. Those behaviors may reflect a sensory-based need or want, a motor-control deficit, or a motor-planning deficit, or serve as a form of communication for social or nonsocial purposes. This is known as the *primary cause* of the behavior. Behavior often serves multiple functions. For example, it can provide the child with a sensory experience he desires, communicate wants and needs to others, and convince others to give the child what he seeks. All of these are very strong motivators for using behavior, which can make change difficult. See chapter 8, Behavioral Intervention Techniques.

Obtaining Behaviors
- Communication
    - Attention
    - Object, Activity, Task
- Internal/Systemic
    - Sensory
        - Productive
        - Nonproductive
    - Systemic

Avoidance/Escape Behaviors
- Communication
    - Attention
    - Task, Activity, Object
- Internal/Systemic
    - Sensory
    - Systemic/Visceral

What Promoted the Behavior? The Antecedent

How do we know whether a child is trying to obtain or avoid something? Behaviors seldom occur in isolation. They are connected to activities or events within their environment, which set the stage for the behavior and give us valuable clues to the purpose they serve.

When beginning to analyze a behavior, it is important to look at its antecedent. What happened *immediately* before the behavior? This may be a task that was introduced, attention given to another child, a loud or abrupt noise, physical contact with another child or an adult, or the cessation of an activity, just to name a few. Knowing what the event or antecedent was will give us clues to the cause of the behavior and help us identify whether the behavior is aimed at obtaining something or avoiding something.

ABC's of Analyzing Behaviors

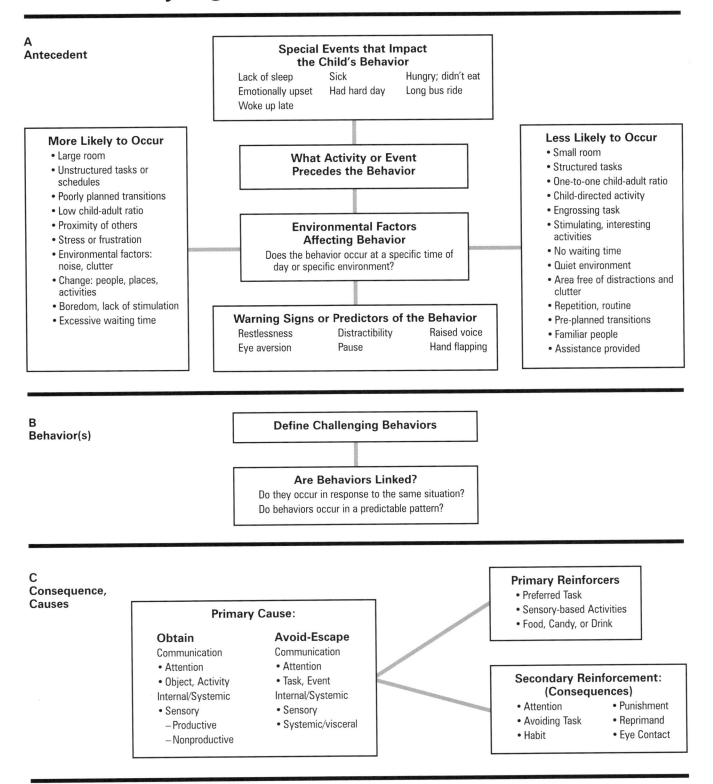

**A
Antecedent**

**Special Events that Impact
the Child's Behavior**

Lack of sleep   Sick   Hungry; didn't eat
Emotionally upset Had hard day   Long bus ride
Woke up late

More Likely to Occur
- Large room
- Unstructured tasks or schedules
- Poorly planned transitions
- Low child-adult ratio
- Proximity of others
- Stress or frustration
- Environmental factors: noise, clutter
- Change: people, places, activities
- Boredom, lack of stimulation
- Excessive waiting time

**What Activity or Event
Precedes the Behavior**

**Environmental Factors
Affecting Behavior**
Does the behavior occur at a specific time of day or specific environment?

Warning Signs or Predictors of the Behavior
Restlessness   Distractibility   Raised voice
Eye aversion   Pause   Hand flapping

Less Likely to Occur
- Small room
- Structured tasks
- One-to-one child-adult ratio
- Child-directed activity
- Engrossing task
- Stimulating, interesting activities
- No waiting time
- Quiet environment
- Area free of distractions and clutter
- Repetition, routine
- Pre-planned transitions
- Familiar people
- Assistance provided

**B
Behavior(s)**

Define Challenging Behaviors

Are Behaviors Linked?
Do they occur in response to the same situation?
Do behaviors occur in a predictable pattern?

**C
Consequence,
Causes**

Primary Cause:

Obtain
Communication
- Attention
- Object, Activity
Internal/Systemic
- Sensory
  - Productive
  - Nonproductive

Avoid-Escape
Communication
- Attention
- Task, Event
Internal/Systemic
- Sensory
- Systemic/visceral

Primary Reinforcers
- Preferred Task
- Sensory-based Activities
- Food, Candy, or Drink

**Secondary Reinforcement:
(Consequences)**
- Attention   • Punishment
- Avoiding Task   • Reprimand
- Habit   • Eye Contact

Figure 4.1   ABC's of analyzing behaviors

Environmental Influences on Behavior

Behavioral responses change depending on the environment. The same task presented in a different environment may result in a completely different response. For example, a child may have no difficulty following directions in a one-to-one situation, but in gym class can't seem to focus, and instead acts out and gets in trouble. Many environmental factors serve as catalysts to problematic behaviors (see Table 4.1). Unstructured tasks can seem endless to the child who will easily get frustrated or overwhelmed. Noisy or cluttered environments can overstimulate or disorganize the child; frequent changes in activities, excessive waiting times, crowded rooms, and boring tasks tend to increase the probability that problematic behaviors will occur.

Altering environmental factors to make the behavior *less likely* to occur is often all that is needed to change behaviors. See chapter 7, Environmental Intervention Techniques, and appendix E.

Table 4.1
Environmental Factors That Impact Behavior

Behaviors Are More Likely to Occur	Behaviors Are Less Likely to Occur
▪ Large room	▪ Small room
▪ Unstructured tasks or schedules	▪ Structured tasks
▪ Poorly planned transitions	▪ One-to-one child-adult ratio
▪ Low child-adult ratio	▪ Engrossing task
▪ Proximity of others	▪ Stimulating, interesting activities
▪ Stress or frustration	▪ No waiting time
▪ Environmental factors: noise, clutter	▪ Quiet environment
▪ Change: people, places, activities	▪ Area free of distractions and clutter
▪ Bored, lack of stimulation	▪ Repetition, routine
▪ Excessive waiting time	▪ Pre-planned transitions
	▪ Familiar people
	▪ Assistance provided

Note. The environmental factors identified above are to be used as a general guide to assist your observation skills. No two children are the same. Environmental factors that diminish one child's challenging behavior may actually increase another's. Individualize a list for each child and each challenging or difficult-to-manage behavior.

Source: Murray-Slutsky and Paris 2000. Used by permission.

Events That Affect the Child

Special circumstances that affect the child internally (internal systemic) also set the child up for negative behavior. These events cannot be ignored. When a child acts out of the ordinary or is having an unusually hard day, it is important to question whether something unusual is affecting him or her. The child may not have slept well, was up late the night before, spent the night at someone else's (friend's/relative's) home, did not eat breakfast or lunch, is ill, or is emotionally upset. Even the weather can throw off some children. Some events occur daily and can affect the child, such as a long car or bus ride or family unrest. Adults involved with the care of the child (parents, teachers, therapists, and caretakers) must communicate with each other when an unusual circumstance occurs that might have an impact on a child's behavior.

Analyzing Behavior Checklist

The following analyzing behavior checklist will help guide you through the problem-solving process. Each of the areas is explained throughout this and subsequent chapters. Using the layering system, each chapter will build upon the other until you have the skills needed to completely analyze problem behaviors and design an intervention program. Chapters 11 and 12 will synthesize this knowledge as you utilize the checklist and the behavioral analysis worksheet (in appendix D) to sort through the behavioral chaos of two case studies.

Analyzing Behaviors Checklist

Behaviors

Define the behavior(s):

Are the behaviors linked?

    Do they stem from the same cause?

    Do the behaviors occur in a predictable pattern?

If both answers are no, then each behavior must be addressed separately.

Priority for change: Is it:
- ☐ Harmful to self and others
- ☐ Destructive
- ☐ Disruptive to others or interferes with learning
- ☐ Socially unacceptable

Antecedent

When does the behavior occur?

In what environments does the behavior occur?
- ☐ Size of room:
- ☐ Structured or unstructured tasks:
- ☐ Adult-child ratio:
- ☐ Environmental factors—noise level, clutter:
- ☐ Time of day—morning or evenings, during transitions:
- ☐ Other:

Characteristics of the activity, if it occurs during activities:

What activity or event preceded the behavior?

Are there any special events that impact the child's behavior?
- ☐ Recent illness
- ☐ Lack of sleep
- ☐ Emotional episode (family dispute)
- ☐ Other:

Warning signs the behavior is about to occur:
- ☐ Restlessness
- ☐ Eye aversion
- ☐ Distractibility
- ☐ Frustration
- ☐ Pause

☐ Raised voice

☐ Self-stimulation or repetitive pattern. Describe:

☐ Other:

Primary Cause

☐ Is the child trying to *communicate* that he wants to *obtain* something?

- Is he trying to obtain attention?

- Is he trying to obtain an object, activity, need or want?

  ▪ Is his communication acceptable?

  ▪ Is his communication unacceptable?
    If Yes, you must address communication strategies.

☐ Is he trying to *obtain* something internal/systemic—in other words, *sensory*?

- Is it productive to meet a need?

  ▪ Is the way he is meeting the need acceptable?

  ▪ Is it effective?

  ▪ Is it nonproductive?

☐ Is he trying to *communicate* that he wants to *avoid* something?

- Is he trying to avoid attention, people, situations, negative attention, and transitions?

- Is he trying to avoid a task, object, or activity?

  ▪ What are the results of the task analysis?

    Skills analysis?

    Emotional analysis?

  ▪ Why is he trying to avoid the task?

    ☐ Task too difficult

    ☐ Task not stimulating/challenging, or task is boring

    ☐ Difficulty adjusting to transition

    ☐ Dislikes task

    ☐ Lacks self-confidence

    ☐ Fears task

    ☐ Avoids task due to sensory aspect

    ☐ Task has no meaning

☐ Is he trying to *avoid* something internal/systemic, in other words, something *sensory*, either avoiding sensory input from his environment or internally?

- Is he overstimulated, overaroused or having difficulty processing sensory input?

  ▪ Is he trying to avoid a specific type of sensory input? Auditory, vestibular, tactile, visual, olfactory (smell)?

  ▪ Is the environment causing it?

- Is he having an internal reaction, such as an illness, feeling hot, hunger, or need to toilet?

Consequences

What happened after the behavior?

What predicts the behavior? Include activities that promote the behavior and warning signs.

Are there any consequences to the behavior? If so, what?

What is primary cause of the behaviors?

What is the primary reinforcer to the behavior?

What are secondary reinforcers?

Summary—Action Plan

Define the behavior(s) needing change.

What are the functions the behavior serves?

Do you plan to stop, alter, limit, or treat the underlying cause, or ignore the behavior?

What environmental changes are needed?

What is reinforcing the behavior?

Define the behavior you want to occur.

What skills do you need to give or teach the child?

What sensory issues must you address?

Do you need a sensory program?

Sensory diet? If so, what?

Sensory integration treatment?

Do you need to address communication strategies?

How will you address this?

What environmental changes are needed?

What will be your reinforcers?

What behavioral strategies will you use?

Do you need to refer to other professionals? OT, PT, ST, behavioralists, or sensory integrative therapists?

Defining Behaviors

We cannot change a behavior unless we can define it in concrete, objective terms. It must be observable to all, and it must be something that occurs more than once (repeatable). Environmental factors in which the behavior specifically occurs should also be noted. Everyone who deals with the child must understand what behavior is to be changed and agree with the definition of the problem. Aggression and disruptive or off-task behaviors are general terms that are neither objective nor observable by everyone. Instead, behaviors may be described as "Throwing objects off his desk," "During writing tasks she cries or runs out of the room," "In class he gets his pencil box out and plays with the objects in the box."

Behaviors are often *linked* as in a chain, making it difficult to know what behavior to list. All of the behaviors serve the same purpose but may occur in a different order each time. Defining one behavior does not capture the essence of the problem; in fact, it is the combination of all of the behaviors that creates the problem. It is important to list all behaviors linked to a single problem.

Adam is disruptive in his class because of his constant movement. He hates to sit in his chair. Instead, he stands next to his desk pushing his arms into the desk and lifting his feet. When he sits in his chair, his feet are often on the table. He rocks his chair forward and backward and frequently falls out of it. He stretches his arms high over his head or locks his hands together stretching and swaying side-to-side. All of these behaviors appear to have the same purpose. The behavior might be defined as proprioceptive-vestibular seeking, used during seated activities to keep his arousal level up. His behaviors are sensory-seeking (obtaining) and make it easier for him to attend and complete his work (productive). However, the therapists working with him would be the only ones who would understand what behaviors had been defined. A more objective, observable definition might be: "Adam uses extraneous body movements during seated activities in the classroom and displays out-of-seat behavior—Behaviors include: . . . "

Nicholas flees a situation when he becomes tired or does not want to do the particular activity. If pressed to continue, he bangs his head. If still pressed to continue, he throws himself to the floor and begins to thrash about. These behaviors are linked and predictable. The inappropriate behavior can be defined as running away from tasks or head banging. The purpose it serves is both task avoidance (communication) and internal systemic avoidance (sensory).

Warning Signs

Warning signs are important cues that the behavior is about to be displayed. People who know the child well can often help identify the warning signs. The child may start to whine, become restless, lose eye contact, or become distracted or disorganized. Increased respiration (breathing) rate, vocalizations, and grinding of teeth can be outward signs of increasing stress and signals that problem behaviors are not far away (see Table 4.2).

Warning signs give us a window of opportunity to intervene before the behavior erupts. The goals of all intervention plans are to teach the child to function without having to resort to the behavior. The best way to do this is to interrupt the problematic behavior, intervene before it occurs, and teach alternative behaviors. If we allow the behavior to occur, we are forced to react to it. *Beginners, who are just learning intervention strategies, often find themselves reacting to challenging behaviors. The intermediate will recognize the warning signs and intervene, teaching alternative coping skills. The advanced practitioner understands the function the behavior serves and designs a program that meets the need, and therefore, eliminates the behavior.*

Table 4.2
Warning Signs or Predictors of the Behavior

Restlessness	Whining
Eye aversion	Hand flapping
Distractibility	Shifting in chair
Frustration	Darting look
Pause	A history of reacting to the task, such as a fine
Raised voice	motor or writing activity

Prioritizing the Need for Change

How important is it to change the behavior? Do you really need or want to change it? This is a very important decision. Many children display so many challenging and difficult behaviors that you could not possibly address all of them. How do you identify what is the most important? The following hierarchy is helpful in prioritizing which behaviors to focus on:

1. Harmful to self or others

2. Destructive

3. Disruptive or distracting

4. Interferes with the ability to learn

5. Socially inappropriate

This hierarchy is influenced by each environmental situation. Adam's out-of-seat behavior is disruptive, which makes it a medium priority for change. However, in the school he attends, his disruptive behaviors place him at risk to be dismissed from the school. The priority for change is urgent due to the environmental situation. Behaviors that are appropriate or insignificant in one situation may be inappropriate or monumental in another. Jumping in place may be appropriate in a physical education class or playtime activity, but this is not a behavior that can be tolerated in a quiet classroom.

Behaviors in which the child harms himself or others are top priority for change. A child who cannot control his aggression or anger, impulsively flees from situations, bangs his head, bites his hands, scratches himself, or pulls out his hair or eyelashes places himself at high risk of injury. The child who physically lashes out, pulling hair, spitting, hitting, or biting, places others at risk of injury.

Destruction of objects or property is also considered a high priority. Behaviors such as throwing objects, swiping small and large objects off desks or bookshelves, or breaking things place the child and those in the immediate vicinity at risk and cannot be tolerated. Destructive tendencies should not be discounted. A young child who throws his own toys when angry will learn that throwing is an appropriate response to anger. It will not stop with toys, but will expand in scope and destructiveness.

Disruptive behaviors disturb others and interfere with their ability to actively participate. These behaviors not only interfere with the child's ability to learn, but often extend to others in the environment. The child who flees when a new task is introduced, hides under a desk in school, calls out in class, is out of or falls out of his seat, or simply fidgets, distracts the teacher and other students. However, all activities that interfere with the child's ability to learn do not necessarily interrupt others. All-consuming preoccupations performed quietly at the desk, such as spinning objects, perseveration on items, or repetitive behaviors or movements can interfere with the child's ability to process and learn.

Children who chew on their shirt, spit, whine, blow their saliva into bubbles, make strange vocalizations, or flap their hands are exhibiting socially inappropriate behaviors that may be targeted for change.

When considering the priority for change, it is important to note that a behavior that may initially appear annoying, and therefore, not a high priority for change, may actually be linked to another behavior that will make it a higher priority.

Vincent would cover his ears when children or babies began to whine or cry, which caused his stress levels to escalate. Covering his ears seemed a low priority for change and was initially thought to be a coping strategy. However, that behavior then became linked to Vincent squeezing the throat of any child or baby making a noise or crying. This linked behavior made the warning sign of covering his ears a higher priority for attention.

Determining What to do With the Behavior: Stop, Alter, Limit, Treat, Ignore

Many people believe that an undesirable behavior should just be eliminated. In some cases this is true. If the underlying cause is not addressed however, purely extinguishing a behavior often results in another, even more undesirable substitute. This is true of behaviors that stem from sensory-based, communication, and postural control deficits. Before electing to purely extinguish a behavior, you must understand the need being served, and carefully weigh if alternative methods should also be used to meet the need.

You have several choices of how to address the behaviors:

1. Stop or eliminate the behavior.

2. Alter the behavior; substitute a more acceptable replacement behavior.

3. Limit the behavior.

4. Treat the primary cause and wait to see if the behavior goes away.

5. Ignore the behavior and do nothing.

High-priority behaviors (that harm the child or others), almost always must be stopped or eliminated. This requires a two-pronged approach in which you develop a program to eliminate the underlying problem at the same time you aggressively intervene to stop the harmful behavior. You can never wait to see if harmful behaviors will go away by treating the underlying cause—a sensory-based or motor control problem. Waiting sets the child and others up for danger. Instead, it requires immediate intervention. A sensory-based or motor control program, implemented at the same time as the behavioral program, will have quicker results than a sensory- or motor-based treatment program or a behavioral program alone.

Behaviors that meet a sensory need are often altered, substituting a more acceptable behavior for the one the child currently engages in. A child who chews on her shirt may be given a chewy necklace or gum to chew instead. A child who flaps his hands when excited may be given a ball or fidget toy and be taught to use it when excited. Because many sensory behaviors are often disruptive, they need to be changed. Eliminating the behavior is often a long-term option, as sensory behaviors are primary reinforcers and reinforce themselves. It requires addressing the underlying sensory issue and the disruptive behavior. The best choice is often to alter the behavior to a more acceptable form that meets the sensory need.

Substituting more acceptable replacement behaviors is often needed when motor control or communication difficulties result in behavioral problems. Rather than throwing a tantrum to avoid difficult work (due to motor difficulties) a child may be taught to request help. Communication-based undesirable behaviors might utilize alternative methods of communication (e.g., sign language, gestures, or pictures) as acceptable replacement behaviors. You may choose to alter a behavior or provide a replacement behavior, *and* treat the underling problem when the behavior is:

1. a higher priority for change,

2. the undesirable behavior is learned, or

3. you cannot wait for the treatment to be effective in order to change the behavior.

Limiting a behavior allows the child to engage in the activity but with rules. The rules may specify when or how the child engages in the activity. For example, with a child who jumps up and down constantly, we may choose to limit the behavior to times when it is socially acceptable to jump or give him specified time on a trampoline or playground.

Many behaviors have an underlying cause that must be treated. For sensory-based behaviors, the underlying sensory issue must be addressed; for communication-based behaviors, the communication issue must be addressed; and for many avoidance behaviors, the underlying motor control must be addressed. The question must be asked: How much of a priority is it to change the behavior? If the behavior is a low priority and you can wait to see the results of intervention, you might decide to treat the underlying issue and wait to see if the behavior disappears. Environmental modifications often fall in this category. If a child is sensory-defensive, overwhelmed by his environment, or is disorganized secondary to environmental issues, the environment may be one of the underlying problems. By modifying the environment the behavioral problems may disappear.

With sensory-based problems another consideration is that problems are often systemic, resulting in more than just one problem. The child's behavioral problems may be so intimately intertwined with his sensory issues that the logical decision may be to address the sensory issues first, before addressing the behaviors. As the child improves, you can choose to address behaviors that are not resolving quickly. For example, Adam's out-of-seat behaviors were definitely proprioceptive and vestibular in nature. He moved continually to alert himself and stay focused. Many of the strategies he used unconsciously throughout his day were effective in obtaining proprioceptive input and increasing his organization, but were distracting to others. Sensory integrative treatments, combined with a sensory diet, quickly diminished his need for these sensory-seeking behaviors. His parents could have elected to treat the underlying problem and see if the behaviors disappeared; however, due to the urgency of his school situation, they chose to limit his behavior within the classroom, while meeting his sensory needs both through his sensory diet and through sensory integrative therapy.

Nicholas, who bangs his head, may be seeking vestibular and proprioceptive inputs. We might use a swing or implement games where he swings, lets go, and crashes to the floor. If the vestibular and proprioceptive inputs attain the same intensity of input that Nicholas gains through head banging, the behavior may be extinguished.

Ignoring a behavior withdraws attention from it. If attention is sustaining the behavior, then ignoring it may extinguish it. By rewarding a desired behavior you may replace it with a more appropriate behavior. For example: If Daniel chooses to whine, you may decide to ignore the behavior and reward him when he is on-task and not whining. If he is seeking attention, the behavior will diminish or disappear if it is not successful. You may also choose to ignore a behavior simply because it is not a high priority for change. Socially inappropriate behaviors, while nice to change, may not be the most important place to focus your time or energy. Ignoring a behavior will not encourage it, and might even diminish it through lack of attention. It is important however, to note that a sensory behavior often reinforces itself, and ignoring it may not alter the behavior.

Consequences to the Behavior

Once the behavior occurs, it is reinforced by either the pleasure derived from the sensory input, the success in meeting the individual's needs, or other consequences. Each of these are reinforcers and contribute to the persistence of the behavior.

It is important to take note of the consequences to the behavior. Often these consequences are attention or negative reactions from the parent or adult, distraction from the task, or success in getting what the child wants. These are only a few of the consequences that become the reason(s) why the child resorts to using the behavior again.

It is important to identify the consequence because it helps define and clarify what the child is trying to obtain or avoid. It also establishes what is sustaining the problematic behavior. Primary and secondary reinforcers sustain a behavior once it has occurred.

Troy has tactile defensiveness that results in avoidance behaviors. He has developed fear of animals, and if he sees a dog or cat he will start screaming and crying, and run away. This has occurred at parks, parties, family gatherings, and public events. His screaming and crying alerts everyone in the area and they run to him, assuming he is severely injured. His parents immediately try to console him. Once he is calm, they try to reason with him about why he should not be afraid. Troy's fears are placing great stress on family members; he dictates where he will and will not go and under what conditions. Troy's sensory issues and anxieties have been addressed, and he has been taught strategies that work for him. However, he refuses to use them because they require effort on his part. He unconsciously chooses manipulative strategies because they are easy, they work, he gets attention, and there are no negative consequences for him. There is no downside or need for him to assume responsibility for his behavior. While his original problem is sensory, and his sensory issues must be addressed, there is a strong behavioral component that must also be addressed in order for him to be successful.

What Is a Reinforcer?

Reinforcers are what encourage or reward behaviors. Almost any behavior has a pay-off or benefit, with some being more obvious than others. For instance, you search the Internet and are rewarded when you find the information you need; you work to receive a paycheck; you complete homework to improve your learning and therefore your grade; you ask questions in order to get answers. *A basic behavioral principle is that any behavior that is followed by a positive reinforcing consequence is more likely to happen again.*

There are many types of reinforcers. Traditionally we think of hugs, kisses, praise, stickers, food, candy, toys, videos, or privileges. However, to find out if something is truly a reinforcer we must determine whether it increases the occurrence of the behavior.

The most important thing to remember is that reinforcers must be individualized. What reinforces one child may not reinforce another. Traditional reinforcers, such as praise from the parent or teacher, or successfully accomplishing a task, may not work. In these cases reinforcers for the specific child must be identified. This can be accomplished by:

- Asking people who know him well for his preferred activity.

- Observing what the child chooses during free time.

- Asking the child his preferred reward.

- Presenting several options and asking the child to choose.

- Presenting various reinforcements and observing how the child responds.

When teaching a new skill, reinforcements should occur after every desired response. As the child's performance improves, reinforcement should be reduced to every second or third response (intermittently). Intermittent reinforcement results in longer-lasting change.

There are two types of reinforcers; primary and secondary. Primary reinforcers are activities or things that are inherently rewarding, such as candy. Secondary reinforcers are activities that are not naturally reinforcing but are associated with pleasure (e.g., praise). The goal is to have the child use the appropriate behavior while receiving intermittent secondary reinforcement.

Primary Reinforcers

Primary reinforcers are activities that are naturally reinforcing. The reward is inherent in the activity. Primary reinforcers are commonly thought of as candy, cookies, snacks, or favorite drinks. They are frequently used in behavioral interventions to reward desired behaviors or responses. Preferred tasks or activities are also used to reinforce desired behaviors. In the case of a child who likes a particular task or activity, the task itself can be a reinforcer for behaviors. If the child enjoys a computer game, the bathtub, a particular toy, or a game or sport, he or she may be encouraged to use the desired behavior in order to obtain it.

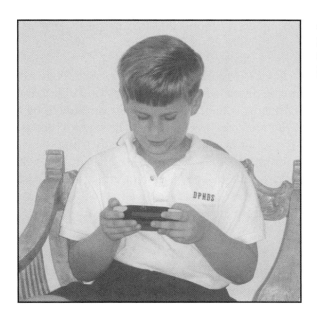

A child who enjoys a particular toy may be encouraged to use the desired behavior in order to obtain it.

Sensory-based activities are less frequently thought of as primary reinforcers, though they are equally, if not more, powerful. Sensory-based activities, if the child prefers and enjoys them, can be the strongest reinforcers of all. The sensory experience can last longer and be more pleasurable to the child, thereby prolonging the reinforcement of the behavior. Because of this, self-stimulatory patterns and obsessive or perseverative behaviors that meet a sensory-based need or want are the strongest and most difficult behaviors to change or extinguish. They are inherently reinforcing for the behaviors.

Lovaas, Newsom, and Hickman (1987), looked at self-stimulatory behaviors within autism. They hypothesized that the self-stimulatory behaviors were primary reinforcers, as the reinforcement was automatically produced by the behavior. Epstein, Taubman, and Lovaas (1985) looked at obsessive behaviors and believed that the obsessive behaviors serve as primary reinforcers. Charlop, Kurtz, and Casey (1990) and Charlop and Haymes (1996) compared use of self-stimulation, echolalia, and perseverative behavior (obsessions) as reinforcers to increase task performance for children with autism. When the child gave a correct response, he or she was allowed to engage in one of the above behaviors for three to five seconds. Interestingly, the authors found that conditions in which these aberrant behaviors were used as reinforcers were more successful than conditions in which food reinforcers were used. Obsessions were associated with the highest percentage of on-task responses and deemed better than self-stimulation or echolalia. No increases in off-task or perseverative behaviors were observed. Obsessions, while individualized to each child, included using numbers, letters, or pictures of the obsession on tokens, or allowing a child to hold the object of obsession briefly.

These studies support the belief that sensory-based, self-stimulatory, and obsessive behaviors are primary reinforcers. Self-stimulatory behaviors, while effective as a reward to enhance learning, increase when reinforced in this manner. It is not recommended to allow a child to engage in self-stimulatory behaviors as a reward for correct behaviors. Brief use (three to five seconds) however, of a child's object of obsession is effective in increasing learning without increasing obsessive behaviors.

A behavior that is followed by a positive reinforcing consequence is more likely to happen again. This behavioral concept applies to the establishment of new replacement behaviors and, unfortunately, is frequently responsible for the persistence of undesirable, challenging behaviors. Favorite activities, tasks, or preferred objects are naturally reinforcing. If the object or activity is obtained successfully through the use of the challenging behavior, the negative behavior is reinforced and will persist. For example, if a child throws a tantrum every time he or she wants a favorite toy or a video, and receives the toy or video, the behavior (tantrum) is reinforced and will continue to be a strategy the child will use in order to get the preferred toy or video. The toy or video is the reinforcer to the tantrum behavior. The adult may be tired and give the child the video in an attempt to calm him or her. However, this only reinforces the frustrating behavior. To make matters worse, the adult may decide to be strong, not giving the child the video when he throws a tantrum three out of four times, then give in the fourth time. This intermittent reinforcement is the strongest method to keep the behavior active.

Secondary Reinforcers

Secondary reinforcers are not inherently pleasing or reinforcing. They have qualities that the child has learned to appreciate. Praise, attention (whether positive or negative), privileges, stickers, eye contact, task avoidance, punishment, reprimands, toys, or activities are a few examples. Praise is the most universal and convenient reinforcer that can be used. Secondary reinforcers, such as tokens, stickers, allowances, or even paychecks, may be used to obtain a primary reinforcer. While a token may be insignificant to a child, if earning ten tokens allows him or her to partake in a favorite activity, the child will quickly learn to value them.

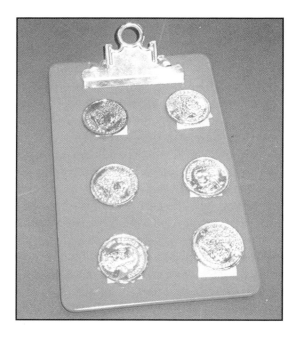

Token boards are a way to teach delayed gratification and are a secondary reinforcer.

A child must learn to appreciate the value of a secondary reinforcer. For some children this comes naturally, while for others it must be taught. To teach a child to value a secondary reinforcer (when he does not naturally appreciate it) it should be provided simultaneously with a primary reinforcer (link the primary reinforcer to the secondary reinforcer). For example:

- While verbally praising a child for a great job (secondary reinforcer) give him or her a small portion of food, a favorite toy, or a pleasurable sensory experience like a hug or applause (primary reinforcer). The praise will increase in value to the child. Gradually diminish the use of the primary reinforcement, while leaving the praise.

- Determine the primary reinforcer the child wants to work for, possibly time watching TV, a favorite video, or a special trip or outing. Cut out a picture of the activity and place it on the token board. Determine the number of tokens that he or she needs to earn for the desired activity (primary reinforcer) and the desired behavior that will earn the tokens. Every time the child earns a token (secondary reinforcer); connect it verbally to the activity he or she is working for (primary reinforcer).

- With a child who values attention, link praise to the attention. Gradually decrease the attention and continue with the praise. For example, when a child does the desired behavior or completes a task as desired, go over to the child, make direct eye contact and let him or her know with enthusiasm exactly what you liked (praise). The child will soon feel great with just the words.

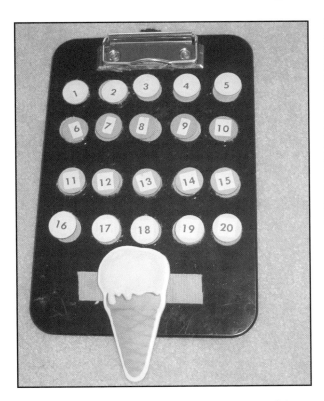

A picture of the item the child is working for is placed on the token board.

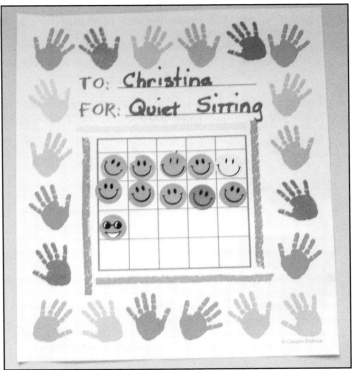

Stickers are given to the child as a reward for sitting quietly. Attention is given to on-task behavior.

Learned Behaviors

When a child responds in the same way to a particular event, the behavior becomes learned. It originates because of a need (primary cause) and is reinforced by either primary or secondary reinforcers. The child continues to engage in the behavior because it meets his needs and it's reinforced, but also because the behavior is learned. It becomes an established behavior, repeated every time the event occurs. Even those behaviors that originated due to a sensory need, a lack of motor control or the ability to plan and sequence a task (motor planning), or those that develop out of a need to communicate something, persist because of their original success in meeting the need. However, they are also learned behaviors. Unless the learned behavior is directly addressed, the behavior may persist long after the primary cause of the behavior (or underlying problem) has been met. Behavioral problems may linger behind, interfering with the child's skill development, long after the underlying problem has been remediated. Addressing the child's learned behavior at the same time as the underlying problem (primary cause), whether sensory, motor, or communication, alleviates the need to address lingering behavioral issues and helps establish healthy coping strategies.

Summary: Important Concepts

- Behaviors can serve multiple functions.

- Analyzing behaviors requires identifying the ABC's of behavior—(A) antecedent and warning signs, (B) defining behavior, and (C) consequence.

- Any behavior that is followed by a positive reinforcing consequence is more likely to happen again.

- The need to change behaviors is prioritized based on the degree of harm or interference with learning.

- Behaviors may be stopped or eliminated, altered, limited, ignored, or the underlying cause treated to see if the behavior goes away. This choice is based on the prioritization for change rating scale and the underlying cause.

- To be rid of a problematic behavior:

  - link the desired response to a primary reinforcer,

  - teach the child to appreciate the reinforcing value of the secondary reinforcer, linking the secondary reinforcer to the primary reinforcer,

  - fade the use of the primary reinforcer,

  - use the secondary reinforcement intermittently, and

  - ignore the undesirable behavior.

- Behaviors that are repeated are learned and may become an established way of responding to a specific situation.

Sensory: Analyzing the Behavior   5

Behaviors are provoked by situations and events in children's lives. These behaviors stem from either a need to obtain something they want or to avoid something they do not want. To complicate the picture, behavior can serve multiple functions: to provide children with a sensory experience they need or desire; to communicate their wants and needs to others; to convey hunger or other needs; or to convince others to give them what they seek. It may be difficult to tease out the primary cause or even the primary and secondary reinforcers, but that is precisely what needs to be done to formulate a plan for changing undesirable behaviors.

Forming a Hypothesis or Theory and Developing a Plan

Obtain

Analyzing the purpose that the behavior serves is the first step in formulating a working hypothesis. Is it sensory? Here is a look at sensory-obtaining and avoidance behaviors.

Obtaining Behaviors

Obtaining behaviors may be provoked by a situation or event or may evolve out of a need. That need may be to obtain a certain sensory or motor experience or activity that provides the child with a pleasurable feeling (internalized/systemic); to communicate a need or want to someone; or simply to obtain attention (social/communication).

Obtaining Behaviors — Internal/Systemic Sensory-Based Behaviors

Sensory-based behaviors are provoked by one or more situations (or needs) and then often are maintained by two or three reinforcers. Sensory feedback or sensory experiences are among the most potent primary reinforcers. They are inherently pleasing to the child, and therefore, perpetuate the behavior.

The child who is hyposensitive or underresponsive to sensory input will often display sensory seeking or obtaining behaviors. The components of sensory-based behaviors stem from the various senses: vestibular or balance system, proprioceptive or position sense, the somatosensory or touch-pressure system, taste (gustatory system), hearing (auditory system), or smell (olfactory system). A child who enjoys the sensory experiences in any one of these systems may exhibit behaviors that derive input from those systems.

Movement of the head or vibration to the face stimulates the *vestibular system*. Vestibular input contributes to the sense of balance, head control, eye gaze, coordination of the two sides of the body, muscle tone and posture, and contributes to the child's core stability, emotionally and physically. Vestibular inputs have the power to wake up the system. Typically developing children often go through phases in which they seek

Analyzing "Obtaining" Behaviors

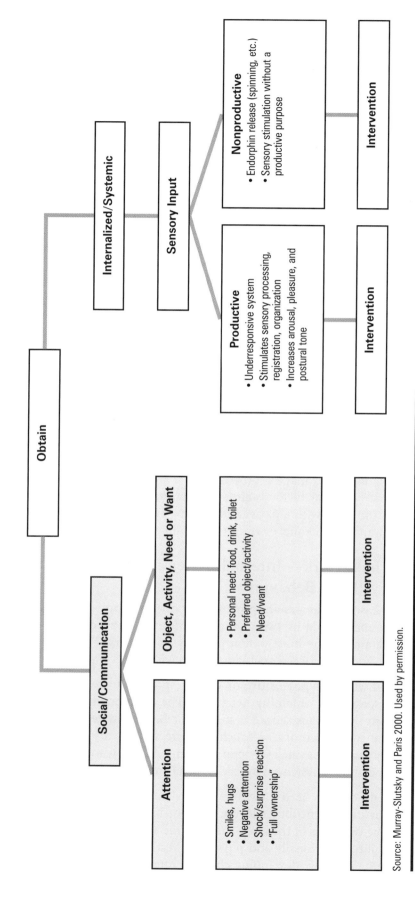

Source: Murray-Slutsky and Paris 2000. Used by permission.

Figure 5.1   Analyzing obtaining behaviors

vestibular inputs. They may use a Sit and Spin®, spin in circles until they fall down dizzy and giggling, or perform rolling games and cartwheels. Both children and adults may rock in their seats or kick their legs to stay awake in classrooms or meetings.

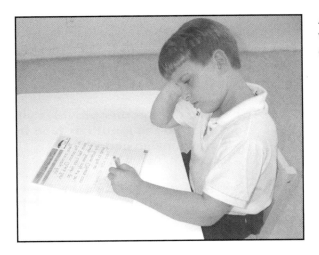

A child with low muscle tone will tend to slump in his chair or over a table.

Hyposensitive or underresponsive children may seek vestibular-based input for its ability to increase arousal levels; for the pleasure of the vestibular input; to stimulate their ability to process by increasing their attentional mechanisms; and/or for improved organization of behaviors. Children who have difficulty sitting still or staying in their seat may need to keep moving in order to function. They may crave intense movements such as bouncing on furniture, turning in a swivel chair, running, jumping on a trampoline, assuming upside-down positions, or swinging high and for long periods. While some children appear overactive, others appear underactive. These children may have low muscle tone (a loose and floppy body); tend to slump or sprawl in a chair or over a table; constantly lean their head on their hand or arm; sit on the floor with their legs in a "W," or fatigue easily. They may have difficulties with gross motor skills and frequently trip or fall, appearing clumsy, especially at sports. They may have difficulty using two hands together for tasks such as cutting or holding a page steady when writing, or they may not have an established hand dominance and continue to write or color with either hand after the age of four or five.

Obtain

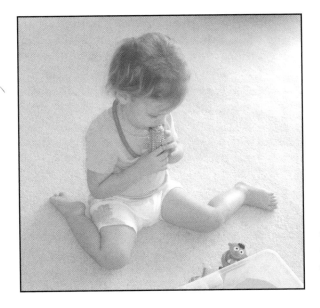

W-sitting is frequently used by children with low muscle tone.

Underresponsive children who want or need to wake up their systems may try rocking, jumping, pacing, or spinning. Children will also use singing and humming for the vibratory sensation it yields. They may seek vibration to the face via a vibrator or a vibrating toothbrush, or press a battery-operated toy to their face.

More aggressive forms of vestibular stimulation often occur when the child is frustrated, disorganized, or overstimulated. The child may throw himself to the floor, thrash in tantrums or head bang. These aggressive behaviors are believed to trigger the release of endorphins that dull pain and can give an internal pleasure response.

Obtain

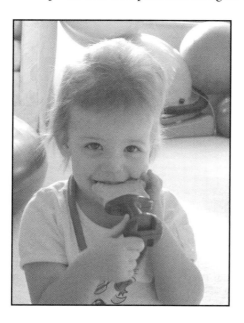

The vibrating teether provides vibratory sensation to the mouth or face for the underresponsive child.

The *tactile system* involves the skin and mouth. Children underresponsive within the tactile system have such a high threshold for registering sensory information that they do not receive adequate information from their hands, legs, and mouth. They must repeatedly touch and feel objects (or mouth objects) to learn about their weight, texture, and shape. They are often very "touchy-feely," touching everything in sight, running their hands across surfaces, bumping into and touching others, taking things from other children, or mouthing objects or their shirt. Although they may touch everything, manipulation of smaller objects may be difficult for them. They will need to look at their hands when they dress, and have a difficult time with zippers or buttons. They may learn to put their socks on in unusual ways. They may not notice when they are dirty, messy, drooling or disheveled-looking. They are unable to tell what is in their hands without looking and will have difficulty getting things out of their desk without pulling everything out. They may be a safety hazard, unaware of impending danger; or show little reaction to pain from scrapes, bruises, cuts, or shots. They may hurt pets or other children, appearing to be without remorse, when actually they cannot comprehend the pain others feel. They may also be afraid of the dark.

This type of processing problem interferes with children's ability to use their fingers, hands, tongue, lips, mouth, legs, or body for skilled discriminatory tasks. They may have difficulty isolating their fingers to show how old they are, holding and controlling a pencil or utensil, writing without looking at their fingers, or using scissors. They may be uncertain of how to move their tongue, lips, or cheeks; or have difficulty speaking, articulating sounds, eating a variety of foods, or blowing whistles. They may mouth objects or use their mouth as a third hand to help with fine motor tasks. Their gross motor skills are often awkward and uncoordinated, and they may have difficulty with age-appropriate skills. In older children this often affects such skills as riding a bike or skating.

Behaviors that arise to stimulate this system include shaking their hands, excessively rubbing or biting the skin, picking at the skin, mouthing toys and objects, bumping or touching others, preferring excessively spicy or sweet foods, or eating only a few select items.

The *proprioceptive system* involves our awareness of where we are in space and in relation to our environment. It is the system through which we perceive deep-touch or pressure, resistance to movement, and the calming effect of those two sensations. The proprioceptive system is one that perceives the benefits of a massage or a heavy exercise workout that relaxes us and aids us in self-regulation.

Proprioception is defined as the cornerstone of sensory integrative intervention (Roley et al. 2001). Its input has the capacity to affect arousal levels, specifically by calming and organizing a person who is overstimulated. It also exerts a regulatory influence over other sensory systems, helping to calm and organize the nervous system when overresponding to touch (tactile) or movement (vestibular) sensations. Activities rich in proprioception are key components to sensory integrative intervention programs due to its effect on arousal levels, body awareness, modulation of vestibular and tactile input, and the increased feedback a child receives from his motor movements.

Obtain

Proprioception is obtained when there is joint traction or compression. This occurs when weights are used or the child uses his own body weight as resistance, as in climbing on playground equipment, such as monkey bars, ladders, ropes or walls; wheelbarrow walking; or tug-of-war games. Behaviors that arise to stimulate this system may include running, jumping, crashing into objects, climbing on furniture and jumping, and rough-housing. Problematic behaviors that may arise from a need or desire to stimulate this system include: pinching, fisting, shaking, or stiffening of the hands or extremities, overfocusing with the eyes, biting, or head banging. Symptoms of difficulties within this system include: difficulty grading pressure (too hard or too light); a tendency to break things, bump into things or people; stamping or slapping feet when walking; poor body awareness; a preference for having shoes or belt tightly fastened; or chewing on objects like shirts, collars, pencils, toys, or gum. These children may have poor posture, slump in their chairs, lean on their hands when working at their desk, be unable to stand on one foot, avoid participating in everyday movement activities or new physical challenges, or may be shy in new situations.

Hyposensitivities to proprioceptive input, decreased body awareness, and poor coordination can lead to motor-planning difficulties. Children may have difficulty conceptualizing, organizing, and sequencing unfamiliar movements and tasks. When they learn a task they cannot generalize it to other situations or environments. Adults become frustrated because they know the child has learned the information or task but cannot remember how to do it or can only do it one way or in one place (at home or school). These children may have difficulty planning and executing motor tasks such as tucking in their shirt, keeping it straight and buttoned, putting on glasses, figuring out how to position their bodies to get their feet in socks, arms into a shirt, or to get into a coat when someone is holding it. They may resist new activities and situations, controlling when, where, and how activities are completed.

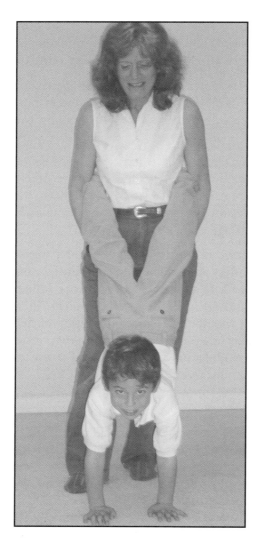

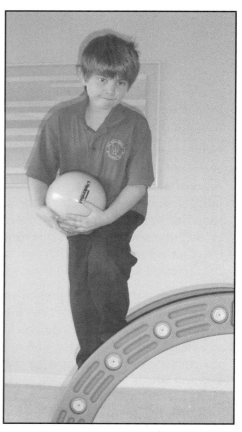

Weight-bearing activities provide proprioceptive input, which helps the child calm himself and helps with body awareness.

A weighted medicine ball provides heavy exercise to improve proprioception, aids in calming, and gives better body scheme.

Children who exhibit these types of behaviors may do well with heavy exercise, deep massage, joint compression techniques, and weight-bearing activities. The proprioceptive input that these types of techniques offer will aid these children in calming themselves and give them a better awareness of their body scheme and how they relate to their environment.

For characteristics of hyporesponsiveness to tactile and proprioceptive sensory input and intervention strategies, refer to appendix A.

The *auditory system* responds to sounds and vibrations. The hyposensitive or underresponsive child may display behaviors that stimulate this sense, such as humming, singing, whistling, talking or jargoning (babbling) nonstop, and vocal play. More problematic forms of auditory stimulation behaviors include shrieking, grinding the teeth or bruxing, flicking the ears, or pulling at the ears. These children may also display difficulties with auditory-language processing, seeming unaware of the source of sounds; looking around to see where the sound came from; not responding when spoken to;

ignoring someone who calls their name; looking at others before responding; having trouble listening or remembering what they were to do; frequently asking people to repeat what they said; or having difficulty discriminating between sounds (bell and ball, boat and bear). They may attempt to increase their auditory processing time by repeating what is said to them. They may also have problems putting thoughts into words, reading out loud, or speaking and articulating clearly. Speech may actually improve after they experience intense movement such as running, jumping, or swinging.

Because of the close association between the auditory and vestibular systems, problems with auditory processing are often seen in combination with problems within vestibular processing and vice versa. When systems that are closely linked, such as vestibular and auditory, are worked together in therapy, there are often improvements in both systems.

Obtaining Behaviors — Internal/Systemic
Sensory Behaviors
Productive or Nonproductive

The question to consider when addressing obtaining sensory behaviors is whether the behaviors are productive or nonproductive and, if productive, are they acceptable?

Productive Sensory Behaviors

Productive, sensory-seeking behaviors are those in which the child consciously or unconsciously seeks to obtain sensory experiences that serve a purpose or meet a basic sensorimotor need. Usually the child is underresponsive (hyposensitive) to sensory input and needs enhanced sensory input in order to improve the processing, registration, or organization of sensory information. Individuals may also use sensory-seeking behaviors to sustain their arousal levels and stay awake and alert, or to increase their awareness of their body. *Productive sensory-obtaining behaviors are the keys to self-regulation.* It is through analyzing what sensory information the child is seeking that we can unlock the mystery to what will help the child obtain self-regulation.

Children inherently seek out information that helps them make sense of their world. Children who are underresponsive to touch or to knowing where their arms and legs are moving (proprioceptive information) may play too hard with others or prefer "crashing" games. This is productive in that it helps these children process their environment and better interpret information coming in from the environment. Children with low postural tone and low arousal levels may run around, appear hyperactive, jump up and down, and flap their hands. These behaviors may serve a sensory-motor purpose to increase the child's arousal levels and postural tone. It may help them function more effectively in their environment, while simultaneously giving them a pleasurable feeling. These children may seek swinging, jumping, or crashing activities as a method of self-regulating elevated stress levels. If the hyperactivity leads to disorganization or to deterioration in behavior, it may be nonproductive and require intervention.

Are these productive sensory behaviors acceptable? While these behaviors are productive, it is important to realize that they may not be considered desirable or socially acceptable. Another concern is that the behavior may serve a purpose but may be ineffective in meeting that purpose. For example, children with low arousal levels who are underresponsive to vestibular input may move about and fidget constantly to keep their arousal levels high. They may not know how to use constructive strategies effectively, may need heavy work, and may not know how or what to do in order to benefit. They may wander aimlessly on the playground, play in a corner by themselves, or simply run.

However, this behavior may actually disorganize them, making the behavior ineffective. The behavior also may be appropriate in one environment and not in another. Running can be appropriate at playtime, but not in the classroom setting.

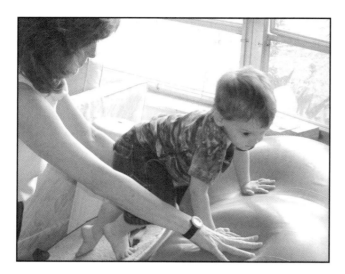

Children who are under-responsive to touch or knowing where their bodies are moving may prefer resistive climbing or "crashing" games.

Obtain

When determining if a productive sensory-based behavior is acceptable, you must first identify the purpose it serves, then its effectiveness in meeting the child's need. If it is ineffective, how do you need to change it, or what can you teach the child that is appropriate to meet his needs effectively? If it is effective, but not acceptable, what is the priority for change? Is the behavior harmful to the child or others, destructive, disruptive, or socially unacceptable? Even a productive sensory behavior can be a priority for change and unacceptable. A child may rock in his chair and fidget to effectively keep his arousal level up and his attention on the teacher. However, it can be unacceptable if it distracts his classmates and interrupts the teacher. This behavior becomes an even higher priority for change if his disruptive behavior may result in the child being asked to withdraw from the class.

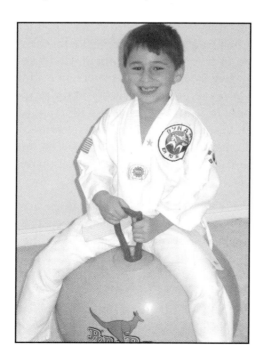

A Hop-n-Bounce or Pon Pon™ provides constructive proprioceptive and vestibular input to the sensory-seeking child.

When looking at intervention strategies, these factors become critical in effectively analyzing and designing a remediation program. *Elimination of an undesirable behavior that serves a productive sensory need, without addressing that need, results in the emergence of another behavior.* Often the new behavior may be even more unacceptable than the original. A child who needs additional sensory input can productively receive it on the playground through climbing, running, jumping, tumbling, and crashing. These sensory-seeking behaviors are both productive and acceptable. These same behaviors, while serving a productive purpose, are undesirable within a classroom situation, and alternative methods must be provided. These same behaviors, while serving a productive purpose, are undesirable within a classroom situation, and alternative methods must be obtained. Equipment such as the Hop-n-Bounce, Pon Pon™, and inflatable seat cushions have been successfully integrated into classroom situations.

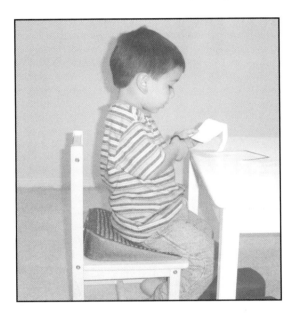

Inflatable seat cushions can provide constructive vestibular input and can position the child correctly for work.

Nonproductive Sensory-Obtaining Behaviors

Nonproductive, sensory-seeking behaviors often are characterized as self-stimulation behaviors that create a pleasurable sensory experience for the child. It has been posited that the self-stimulation results in an endorphin release that in turn causes an internal pleasure response. Often these behaviors are viewed as disruptive to others, socially inappropriate, and interfere with the child's ability to learn or interact with others. Examples of nonproductive sensory behaviors may include rocking, self-spinning, and jumping. In autism and other disorders, these behaviors may include head banging, self-biting, or hand-flapping behaviors, among others. A list of sensory-based stereotypic behaviors and their sensory input is provided in appendix C. Intervention for problematic sensory stimulatory behaviors can be found in Table 5.1.

Table 5.1
Modifying Problematic Sensory Stimulation Behaviors

Once a behavior is prioritized for change, modifying or eliminating stereotypic or disruptive behaviors requires a multifaceted approach that addresses the sensorimotor, communication, and behavioral aspects of the behavior.

1. Identify the stereotypic, disruptive, or problematic behavior. Determine if you need to:

   - Stop the behavior

   - Limit the behavior

   - Alter the behavior

   - See if the behavior will extinguish on its own with a sensory-based and communication program

2. Determine what is the sensory stimulation provided from the behavior. Look at:

   - Intensity of the stimulation

   - Duration of the stimulation

   - Frequency of the stimulation

3. When does the behavior occur? What is the need met?

   Communicative, to:

   - Obtain something

   - Avoid or terminate an activity

   - Communicate something

   - Seek something

   Sensory-based, to:

   - Calm self

   - Arouse self

   - Organize self

4. What else keeps the behavior alive?

   - Primary causes

   - Secondary reinforcers or consequences to the behavior

5. Design a program to eliminate the need for the behavior. The techniques that will be used will include:

   - Sensory-based activities

   - Sensory integrative techniques

   - Development of functional skills to eliminate the need for the behavior

   - Environmental modifications

6. Develop communication strategies.

7. Eliminate the behavior through behavior modification techniques.

   - Use physical prompts; then gradually fade all prompts.

Obtain

Basic Intervention Principles—Sensory Obtaining Behaviors

Obtaining Behaviors—Internal/Systemic Sensory Behaviors

There are several key elements in addressing a sensory-based behavior:

Sensory behaviors comprise both sensory and behavior.

- The sensory component is a primary reinforcer.

- The behavior often serves one or more purposes.

- The behavior functions to obtain or avoid either something sensory or communicative.

- The behavior is reinforced by the consequences that occur after the behavior (secondary reinforcers).

If the sensory behavior is productive, effectively meets a need, and is acceptable (not a priority for change), then you do not need to change the behavior.

- Help others understand the purpose to the behavior, become more sensitive and empathetic.

If the sensory behavior is productive (meets the child's needs), but is not acceptable (a priority for change), then you must help the child change the behavior.

A nonproductive behavior with a priority for change should be changed.

Basic guidelines for changing a sensory behavior include:

- Analyze the child's behavior and activities engaged in to determine the sensory need being met.

  1. What are the sensory systems that are underresponsive?

  2. What is the sensory need the child is trying to accomplish when he engages in the activity (e.g., increase arousal, alertness, and awareness of body or hands or the object; or to calm self).

  3. What does the behavior tell you about the sensory system? For example, when a child has poor posture and consistently holds his head up while working at his desk, we might guess the child has an underresponsive vestibular and possibly proprioceptive system.

  4. What is the function served by the behavior, if different from the sensory need? Children may engage in an activity for multiple reasons. You must identify as many as you can. For example, Samantha is presented with a fine motor task that she does not like. She immediately slumps in her chair and slithers to the floor under the table. When repositioned in her chair she continues to fall out. Her tone is normally low and she has difficulty with her posture. She is underresponsive to vestibular and proprioceptive information. However, she is also avoiding a task, making the problem both a sensory and behavioral issue (non-sensory).

- Identify acceptable alternative sensory activities or behaviors that meet the same sensory need, at the same level of intensity of sensory input and same duration and frequency. In the above example, Samantha may be given an inflatable cushion (e.g. Sit and Fit™ or Movin' Sit™ or Sissel™) at school in order for her to bounce and rock in her seat to get the vestibular input needed to raise her muscle tone and postural control for schoolwork.

- Teach, prompt, and reinforce the child to use the alternative method consistently.

- Address the underlying "function" served by the behavior. (See below.)

- Establish routines that address the underlying system and meet the "function" served by the original behavior.

- Use behavioral strategies to stop, alter, limit, or replace the behavior (see chapter 8).

- For more information on establishing routines (sensory diets) refer to chapter 10.

Stopping a sensory behavior that serves a purpose, without meeting that purpose, often results in other, less desirable behaviors.

Intervention for sensory-based behaviors, to address the underlying function served, include:

- Sensory-based activities

- Sensory integrative techniques

- Sensory diets (see chapter 10)

- Environmental and therapeutic modifications to alter arousal levels

- Development of functional skills

- Development of communication strategies

- Implementation of behavioral management strategies (reinforcers for on-task behaviors).

Avoidance Behaviors

Avoidance Behaviors
Internal/Systemic
Sensory Behaviors

Sensory-Based Avoidance

Many of us experience sensory overload during stressful situations. The noise of a television or radio blaring, the overload of being in an overcrowded department store or at a football game can easily send us in search of a quiet place to get away for a few minutes. It is a normal coping mechanism when we feel overloaded and out of control.

Infants and young children will become cranky, not knowing what the problem is or how to deal with it. An overwhelmed child may shut down and fall asleep, thereby avoiding the noise and turbulence of being overstimulated. Others may complain of a headache or stomachache. Some children are overly sensitive; their nervous system registers sensory input more intensely than others, making their nervous systems prone to easy overload. Because of their high sensitivity, it is hard for them to maintain a middle ground, keeping their arousal level and emotions at an appropriate level to function. Their frequent overarousal, or fluctuating arousal levels, result in behavioral responses characterized by problems with attention, focus, registering information in their environment, arousal and self-regulation, and possible shutdown.

"Avoidance" or "Escape" Behaviors

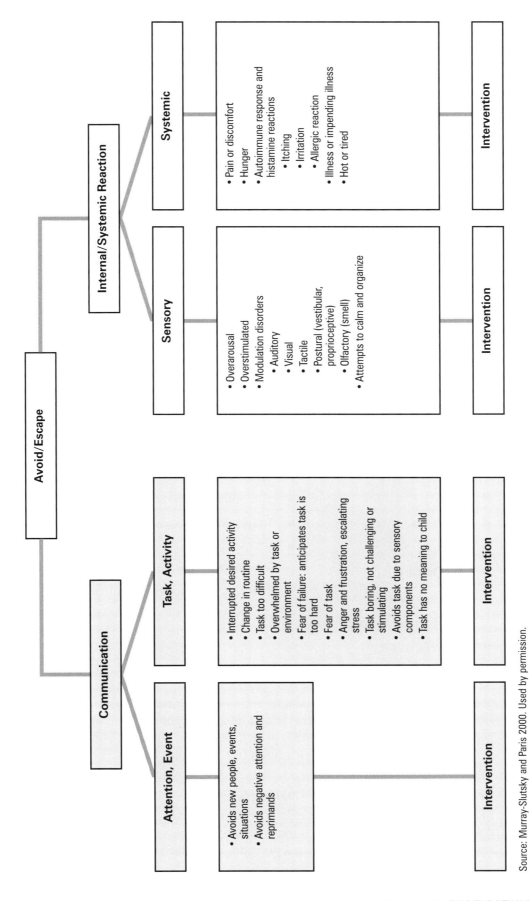

Source: Murray-Slutsky and Paris 2000. Used by permission.

Figure 5.2   Analyzing avoidance or escape behaviors—focus on sensory

Emotional responses are often characterized by stress reactions of fright, flight, or fight, and result in many of the avoidance behaviors we see: sensory avoidance, task avoidance, and attention avoidance behaviors. The core problem is a sensory modulation and regulation problem, which results in the nervous system overresponding to sensory information. The underlying problem is sensory; however, there is often a learned behavior associated with task avoidance. The child has learned to react emotionally not only on the actual activity, but on the anticipation of the event or activity. While helping the child communicate, and addressing the child's task avoidance and attention avoidance issues help, the core problem lies in the fact that the nervous system overresponds to sensory information. This core problem, a sensory modulation and regulation problem, must be addressed either before or at the same time that the avoidance behavior is addressed, in order to treat the primary problem rather than just the symptoms.

Sensory modulation disorder refers to a problem in the capacity to regulate and organize the degree, intensity, and nature of response to sensory input in a graded and adaptive manner. It equates to difficulty with self-regulation and is the inability to effectively regulate arousal levels or match the arousal level to the activity. A modulation disorder interferes with the person's ability to maintain an optimal level of arousal appropriate for the task, and therefore, interferes with the person's ability to effectively meet the challenges encountered every day. A modulation disorder may result from the nervous system being undersensitive (hyporesponsive) to sensory information, resulting in primarily sensory-obtaining behaviors. Oversensitive (hyperresponsive) responses result primarily in sensory-avoidance behaviors. Fluctuating responses characterized by both sensory-avoidance and obtaining behaviors may also be seen.

A child or adult with a modulation disorder would display several of the following difficulties:

- Attention
- Focus
- Registration
- Arousal
    - Overarousal
    - Underarousal
    - Fluctuating arousal
- Self-regulation

- Behavior or emotional responses
- Attending to relevant stimulation
- Responding in an organized fashion
- Using a level of arousal and attention appropriate for the task
- Blocking out irrelevant information

Sensory Overarousal

Sensory-avoidance behaviors characterized by overarousal to sensory information result from a modulation disorder. The behaviors and responses the child displays vary depending on the sensory system that is inefficient. The auditory, visual, tactile, olfactory (smell), gustatory (taste), and proprioceptive-vestibular (balance and posture) sensory systems are the most vulnerable.

Vestibular Hypersensitivities (Defensiveness)

Movement of the head stimulates the *vestibular system*. Movements that are up-and-down, forward-and-backward, rotary, or any combination in between stimulate the vestibular system. Changes in head position, body movement, spinning, turning, lying down, going upside-down, going up and down stairs, or vibration to the face are examples of movement that impact this system.

An overresponsive vestibular system may result in children who display avoidance behaviors. They may dislike playground activities such as swings, slides, or spinning activities; be uncomfortable in elevators or escalators; or experience carsickness. They may be cautious or slow-moving, hesitating to take risks. They may fear falling even when there is no real threat. This fear may extend to walking on raised surfaces such as curbs or stairs, or anytime the feet leave the ground. They may feel threatened with changes of head positions such as being turned upside-down or being tilted forward or backward to have their hair shampooed in a sink. Unexpected movements—the teacher pushing the chair in, a child bumping them in the hall, or a small trip—may elicit a fear, flight, or fight reaction.

For characteristics and intervention strategies for vestibular hypersensitivities, refer to appendix B.

Tactile Hypersensitivities (Defensiveness)

Children who are hypersensitive to tactile or touch information will respond negatively and emotionally to light touch or unexpected touch. Tactile hypersensitivity, also known as tactile defensiveness, causes the protective system to interpret normal contact as threatening. These children are frequently in a state of high alert, ready to react to the slightest invasion. They may get increasingly disorganized, distracted, and irritable by touch. Casual contact, like being brushed, bumped, or touched lightly on the shoulder, or daily contact, such as the strap of the car seat, texture of clothes, having their hair combed or cut, may cause extreme behaviors such as vigorous resistance, fighting or screaming, running away (flight), crying, whining, or passive withdrawal (fright). In some cases, these children may simply avoid the objects and people that distress them. They may walk away from and never get close to the people and things that touch them lightly or unpredictably. They tactfully avoid tactile sensations, pets, people, and activities (finger painting, gluing, playing in the mud) while convincing adults "It's just not their thing."

Tactile hypersensitivity is a sensory processing disorder in which the nervous system overresponds to touch input. The nervous system requires a certain amount of touch information to function. A child's avoidance of touch places the nervous system in a state of sensory deprivation. To avoid this, these children crave deep touch and specific types of input. They crave it and are hungry for sensory input, but must control how, when, and where they get it. They may love firm bear hugs, back rubs, or running a finger lightly across someone's eyelashes. They may repeatedly touch things that they find soothing: have a favorite blanket, run theirs hands repeatedly over things that feel comforting to them, or continually hold an object in their hand. They may be inappropriate in what they touch or how much pressure they exert.

Children with tactile hypersensitivity may be very picky about their clothing, wearing only specific textures, clothing without tags, or shirts without collars. They may be fastidious about cleanliness, not allowing dirt or water to get on them, making sure nothing touches their face, even leaning over when they cry to be sure tears don't touch their face. They may hate haircuts, or having their hair combed, shampooed, or touched. Dentists are particularly threatening, as is brushing their teeth. They may have specific food preferences: eating only one or two specific items, refusing to eat hot or cold foods, or foods with unpredictable lumps (such as vegetable soups or rice pudding). They may walk on their toes, avoid walking barefoot, or avoid walking in sand or grass.

Avoid

These children exert tremendous effort to avoid tactile activities that are threatening to their nervous system; however, their nervous system still quickly overloads to sensory information they can't control. Behaviors seen are characterized by fright, flight, or fight, but they may also display challenging behaviors to "numb" the system, or block out the aversive feeling. They may use deep-touch pressure or proprioceptive input for this purpose and may hit, scratch, or rub themselves or others; push or wrestle with others; run, jump, crash into objects; climb on furniture and jump; roughhouse; put firm pressure with their mouth against others; bite themselves or others; or head bang.

For characteristics and intervention strategies for tactile defensive behaviors, refer to appendix B.

Auditory Hypersensitivity (Defensiveness)

Children may display auditory hypersensitivities (overresponsiveness) with or without auditory-language processing difficulties. They may be unable to pay attention to one voice or sound without being distracted by other sounds, become overwhelmed and disorganized in noisy environments, or become distressed by noises that are loud, sudden, and high-pitched. Even sounds that other people tolerate easily and consider normal may bother them. They may cover their ears, hold their head and ears, hide, run, or become increasingly more active and disorganized. More challenging behaviors may also be displayed, which include grinding their teeth, humming, singing, self-talk, or other steady vocalizations, screaming, or head banging. These challenging behaviors are believed to not only block out the auditory stimuli, but also to trigger chemically mediated responses to calm the child.

For characteristics and intervention strategies for tactile defensive behaviors, refer to appendix B.

Multisensory Processing Difficulties

Children who are susceptible to overstimulation, overarousal, or sensory modulation difficulties may have difficulty with multisensory processing. Each sensory modality (auditory, visual, olfactory, gustatory, tactile, and postural or proprioceptive-vestibular) may easily be registered and processed by the child as a single modality. However, when bombarded with multiple sensory inputs, the child may become overwhelmed, overstimulated, and reactive. Processing of multiple sensory (polymodal) information can be particularly difficult, and the accumulation of information coming in from multiple sensory experiences can trigger undesirable reactions.

In other cases, children may be particularly vulnerable to overarousal of information from one or two senses. Often there is a neurological association between these systems, such as the vestibular system and the auditory system. Tactile defensiveness (hypersensitivity to touch), gravitational insecurities (hypersensitivity to balance and movement), and auditory hypersensitivity are examples of modulation or regulatory disorders seen in specific sensory systems. These disorders may occur in isolation or in combination with other sensitivities. Inconsistencies may be noted as well. The child may be underresponsive to one system and oversensitive to another.

Summary: Sensory Avoiding Behaviors

Those who find themselves overaroused or overstimulated by sensory information, or as a response to sensory integrative dysfunctions like modulation or regulatory disorders, often resort to challenging behaviors as a method of blocking out sensory information to calm their nervous systems. Often, children are not consciously aware that they are experiencing sensory overload. Each child will develop unique coping strategies. A child who is hypersensitive to sound may talk or chatter nonstop to block out other noises in the environment. One who is hypersensitive to touch may obsessively control every aspect of the environment in order to manage the tactile information coming into his or her system, or strike out aggressively in an effort to fight off the overload. Children who are fearful of movement and balance activities may avoid being in crowded rooms, avoid threatening activities, or become aggressive. Children develop unique and often challenging behaviors that help them feel better for the moment but may interfere with their long-term learning and social interaction.

Nonverbal children are particularly at risk of developing challenging behaviors as coping strategies. They may use head banging, biting, grinding of teeth, hiding under objects, or rocking to calm themselves when overstimulated. These methods all are a form of deep-proprioceptive input that neurologically calms the nervous system. Slow, rhythmic movements, such as rocking or head banging, have been known to calm the system and provide a sense of organization through slow vestibular input. Head banging, biting, and other self-injurious behaviors may be used in an attempt to self-calm and self-sedate. The strength of these stimulatory behaviors is believed to trigger the release of endorphins, the body's own pain inhibitors. They are opiate-like substances that numb the system. These challenging behaviors need to be modified into constructive, socially acceptable behaviors that give the child constructive, acceptable methods of meeting sensory-based needs.

Basic Intervention Principles — Sensory Avoidance Behaviors

Avoidance Behaviors — Internal/Systemic Sensory Behaviors

Avoidance due to overarousal, overstimulation, or modulation disorders.

- Identify the elements contributing to overload:

  - Sensory systems

  - Environmental aspects

  - Schedule elements

- Decrease the environmental stimulation (see chapter 7).

- For environmental and therapeutic modifications to decrease arousal levels, refer to appendix E.

- For intervention strategies for specific behaviors, refer to appendix B.

Identify appropriate sensory-based activities effective in calming or organizing the child.

- Teach the child use of alternate activities for calming.

- Guide the child to use alternative methods when needed.

- Teach the child to identify warning signs of sensory overload and use alternate activities early.

- Integrate calming, sensory-based activities into the child's schedule to maintain optimum functioning throughout the day.

- Teach the child to recognize and communicate his feelings.

- For more information on sensory diets, refer to chapter 10.

Remediate the underlying modulation difficulty.

As the underlying sensory-based problem is remediated, systematically increase the child's tolerance for and scope of new activities.

Avoidance Behaviors
Internal/Systemic
Systemic/Visceral

Systemic Avoidance

It takes years for typically developing children to learn how to interpret what they feel inside and to communicate these feeling to adults. Many times, the child describes vague symptoms or discomfort or acts out of the ordinary, but can't locate or identify the cause of the discomfort. The adult struggles to learn what is causing the child to act distressed or out-of-sorts. The child is bombarded with a litany of questions or taken from doctor to doctor until either he starts to feel better or the problem is identified, solved, or disappears.

Children with sensory-related problems experience similar feelings and discomforts. They may feel hot, fatigued, hungry, be in pain, or be generally irritable. Change may be more difficult for them to tolerate, and it may be actually uncomfortable. Very young children and those with sensory-related hypersensitivities may also experience a change inside their bodies and be uncertain of what it is. This internal response may be as simple as hunger, feeling hot, or needing to go to the bathroom; or more intense, like pain or discomfort from an injury. Other possibilities include an illness or impending illness, an allergic reaction to food or something they touched, or a histamine reaction to an insect bite. Still other possibilities include the child who is hyperresponsive to vestibular input and feels the headache, nausea, or dizziness associated with it, or the discomfort felt by those who may be hypersensitive to other sensory modalities.

Children experiencing sensory overload may learn techniques to block out the input or calm their systems; but with internal system reactions, often these children are ineffective in alleviating their discomfort. They may be cranky and inconsolable, frustrated, or escalating in agitation. Challenging behaviors may erupt out of frustration or the disorganization experienced within their systems.

Basic Intervention Principles — Systemic Avoidance Behaviors

Avoidance Behaviors — Internal/Systemic
Systemic/Visceral

Assist parent in differentiating sensory versus medically based concerns.

Look for symptoms that may indicate medically based problems, such as:

- Signs of allergies: irritability, runny nose, watery eyes, circles under eyes, irritation on skin, or rash

- Histamine reactions: flushing, redness, or itching

- Fever

- Pain
- Discomfort or swelling
- Avoiding using an arm or leg

For children with hypersensitivities, look for environmental factors that may be contributing, such as smoke, carpet cleaners, or other unusual smells.

Refer to appropriate medical professional as indicated.

For sensory modulation difficulties, follow steps for sensory-avoidance behaviors as appropriate.

Analyzing Behaviors That Are Not Sensory

6

Behaviors are provoked by situations and events in a child's life. These behaviors stem from either a need to obtain something the child wants or to avoid something he does not want. Behaviors arise to communicate wants and needs to others and may serve as a method to convince others to give the child what he seeks or to allow him to avoid a task or situation. If the behaviors are not triggered by a sensory-based cause, then they are considered simply behaviors that must be addressed.

Obtaining Behaviors — Social/Communication Behaviors

Obtain

Some types of obtaining behaviors are not sensory-obtaining or sensory-seeking behaviors. These behaviors stem from a child's difficulty in communicating his or her needs and wants. We have termed these types of behaviors social/communication obtaining behaviors. Infants and children without the necessary speech and language to communicate their wants or needs often resort to nonverbal methods of communication in order to get their needs met. They may develop an elaborate system of communication that is understood only by people who are intuitive enough to understand them. They may use simple gestures or movements toward the person whose attention they seek or the object of their desire.

Children with good speech and language may also display difficult social/communication behaviors. They may have learned negative strategies that get attention (obtaining behaviors) without communicating. Negative attention-seeking behaviors or full-ownership behaviors are examples of negative obtaining behaviors displayed by children with and without adequate speech and language.

When a child uses problematic or challenging behaviors as a method of communicating, we need to analyze what activity preceded the behavior, as well as the consequence, to discern the primary cause of the behavior.

Obtaining Behaviors
  Social/Communication
  Attention-Seeking Behavior
The child may be seeking positive attention from someone in the environment. The young infant may cry to be picked up; the toddler may want attention, a smile, a kiss, or a hug from a parent. Attention is a powerful reinforcer. Children learn at a very young age how to use their behavior to get what they want. When children scream, adults respond. Children may quickly learn that it is a method to get whatever they want: a glass of water, attention, or any of a variety of objects.

Analyzing "Obtaining" Behaviors

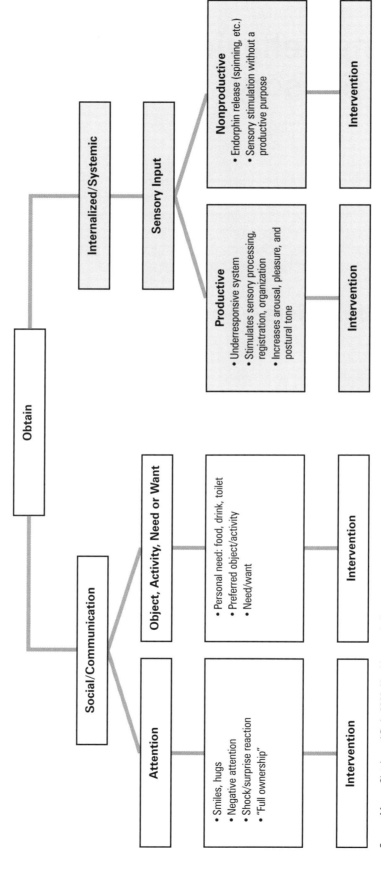

Source: Murray-Slutsky and Paris 2000. Used by permission.

Figure 6.1   Analyzing obtaining behaviors—focus on nonsensory, social communication

Attention of any type can be very rewarding and reinforcing from a child's perspective. Even when the adult intends the interaction to be corrective, it may still be rewarding. For example, a parent may believe that he is admonishing the child for undesirable behavior by explaining why screaming in public is inappropriate. The fact remains that simply allotting attention to the explanation immediately after the behavior occurs gives children the reinforcement for the behavior. Having long conversations with them about how they need to change their behavior; how their aggressive behavior hurt someone else, or any other scenario, may be viewed rewarding. To children it may not matter if it is positive or negative attention, as long as an adult is interacting with them.

Full ownership is the extreme of attention-seeking behaviors, in which children demand the full, undivided attention of the person caring for them or working with them at the time. Parents, therapists, and teachers experience this when a child will not allow them to talk or interact with anyone else. The child may display disruptive behaviors or tantrums to assure the adult's undivided attention. Parents who spend a lot of time with their child often find themselves faced with this situation. They stop to talk to a friend or teacher, or are busy in a grocery store, and suddenly the child is whining or misbehaving. Behavioral strategies are effective in teaching when full-ownership behaviors are not permitted.

In some situations, full-ownership behaviors may be desirable. A child who claims full ownership of an adult will be fully vested in that adult, displaying increased attention, task compliance, and motivation to almost anything the adult asks. This is wonderful when teaching a child or working with a child one-to-one, but is not realistic when the teacher or therapist is faced with a group situation or when a parent has other children to deal with.

Negative Attention-Seeking Behavior

To some children, it may not matter if the attention is for positive or negative reasons, as long as the adult is interacting with them. Just as children may seek positive attention, they can seek negative attention or reactions from people around them. Often parents complain that their child "pushes their buttons." Negative attention singles a child out and provides immediate gratification. It is a powerful reinforcer for some children. It is often the only way they derive attention with the regularity, frequency, and intensity they desire. The negative attention is often not long-lasting, and the frequency of behavior may increase to gain the amount of attention they seek. Children may use negative attention-seeking behaviors, such as mischief, disobedience, or tantrums to get the attention they want. They may begin an activity they know their parents do not want them to engage in, stop long enough to assure their parents have seen them, then continue. They may avert their eyes or not respond to a person speaking to them, forcing the adult to give them one-to-one attention. A child may pinch, bite, slap, or pull the hair of another child to gain attention or may show self-aggression such as head banging to get the attention of an adult.

Cipani (1998) looked at noncompliance in children and its relationship to disruptive and inappropriate classroom behaviors. He believed that obtaining negative attention reinforced the deviant, noncompliant behavior. The child who is noncompliant in class often attracts both the teacher's negative attention and that of others in the class. Rather than the attention coming exclusively from the teachers, it may come in the form of reminders, cajoling, joking, moving closer to the child, or other verbal or nonverbal behaviors (frowns, looks) that follow the noncompliance. Peer reinforcement for acts of noncompliance, usually seen in middle school and high school, can come in the form of laughter, jokes, and other verbal and nonverbal behaviors indicating approval. Noncompliance, as a method of getting negative teacher attention, is seen most frequently with the child who is unable to get attention for positive behaviors such as doing work, sitting quietly, or complying with requests. Cipani cautions that when a child appears to be seeking negative attention through noncompliance, one should verify that the child is capable of complying with the teacher's requests, before embracing a negative attention-seeking hypothesis.

The reinforcement from negative attention often comes through the quality of the consequences. The quality of a negative reaction can be a strong reinforcement to the behavior. A frown, criticism, or a reprimand in a strong voice can be a strong reward. Negative attention often is more strongly and immediately presented than is praise. The sheer strength of the delivery may be what the child responds to and seeks. A surprised or startled reaction often creates a pleasurable experience for children, and they may attempt to recapture it by repeating a behavior. Some children get pleasure from the firmer handling they receive when they act out. Whether they are pulled to stand in the midst of a tantrum, or their arms are grasped by an adult who is trying to prevent the child from hurting himself or others, the deep-proprioceptive input of restraint, the one-to-one attention, and the sharpness of tone that accompany negative attention-seeking behaviors may be enough to ensure that the child will repeat it.

Obtain

This behavioral response of negative attention seeking may be coupled with an underlying sensory issue of underresponsiveness (sensory-obtaining behaviors), creating a vicious cycle in which the child misbehaves, seeks negative attention, and at the same time obtains the desired sensory input. Intervention must address both the sensory and behavioral issues. Intervention strategies addressed in chapter 10 (sensory diets, sensory integrative intervention) need to be incorporated at the same time as intervention for the negative attention-seeking behavior.

Basic Intervention Principles — Attention Seeking Behaviors

Obtaining Behaviors
Social/Communication — Attention-Seeking Behaviors
Give structured positive attention to desired "on-task" behaviors:

- Specify exactly what you liked: "I liked how you raised your hand to ask this question."

- Avoid general praise, such as "good job." General praise leaves room for interpretation; the child may associate it with any behavior.

- Use the child's name; associate it with positive experiences: "John, how nice of you to help Ana."

- Do not inadvertently reward incorrect or inappropriate behavior.

For negative attention-seeking behaviors:
- Ignore the negative attention-seeking behavior.

  - Do not provide secondary reinforcement to the negative behavior. This includes talking about the behavior to the child or to others in front of the child; attending to it; trying to cajole the child; moving closer to the child; etc.

  - Control environmental factors and other persons in the area that may reward the negative behavior.

- Reward the positive, on-task behaviors. Use the child's name and give specific praise.

- If the child does not engage in on-task behavior:
  - Use behavioral strategies to prompt and model desired responses. (See chapter 8, Behavioral Intervention Techniques.)
    - Reward all attempts in the direction of the desired response.

- Look for warning signs that the negative attention-seeking behavior is about to occur:
  - Intervene prior to the negative behavior.
  - Praise desired behavior or prompt desired behavior and reward.

- Be enthusiastic in your praise.
  - Give praise at the same intensity as any negative attention you might have given.
  - Praise more often than you give the negative attention the child was seeking.

- Be consistent.

- Educate all team members, and implement in all environments.

For "full-ownership" behavior—Constructive:
- Determine whether it is constructive. If the child's need for your complete and undivided attention results in increased task compliance, participation, and motivation, then no intervention is required. Full ownership may be helpful when:
  - Working with a child one-to-one, as in therapy, tutoring, or when teaching in a resource room.
  - A parent is at home alone with a child.

- If it is allowed in certain environments, such as those listed above, be specific.

If the full-ownership behavior is undesirable, stifling, or destructive, and the child uses negative attention-seeking behaviors to get your undivided attention:
- Teach the exact situations and environments where it is not allowed.

- Be consistent in enforcing the situations and environments.

- Have the child sit or play in a specified area, while you engage another person in a conversation.

- Give the child something to keep him occupied: a toy, a book, or a game.

- When a child can only sit quietly for ten seconds, have him or her sit and count to ten, or engage briefly in a book or toy. Reward the child for engaging in the diversional activity. Repeat over and over again, gradually increasing the overall amount of time spent waiting. Follow the procedures below to increase waiting time.
  - Reinforce desired behavior. Be specific with your praise: "Anna, I like how you are playing quietly while I talk to your teacher."
  - As you talk, keep your eyes on the child. Look for the warning signs that the child is getting fidgety. Go over and reward desired behavior before the negative behavior occurs.

Obtain

- Use/teach delayed gratification, gradually extending the amount of time the child waits quietly, before rewarding him or her or leaving (see chapter 8, Behavioral Intervention Techniques).

- Keep the child engaged in a diversional task, activity, or game while he or she must wait for you.

Obtaining Behaviors
Social Communication
Behaviors to Obtain a Need or Want, an Object or Activity

Children's behavior often tells us that they want more than just attention. We must always ask ourselves, what are they attempting to communicate? What do they need or want? Sometimes children's behavior communicates strongly what they want, while other times we must search for clues. Analyzing the events that occurred immediately before the behavior (antecedent), the behavior, and the events that occur immediately after (consequences) help us identify what the child is trying to obtain. When Michael runs into class, knocking over children and desks on his way to get to his favorite computer game we clearly know what he is trying to obtain. With Gabriel it's not as obvious. Gabriel had been working quietly when all of a sudden he starts to shift restlessly in his seat, he can no longer concentrate and becomes increasingly agitated, knocking everything off his desk. The teacher knows him and recognizes these behaviors as warning signs that he must go to the bathroom. She learned these warning signs the hard way, from recognizing the consequences—after he had an accident.

Obtain

Children may not be consciously or cortically aware of exactly what they want. They may be hungry and want something to eat or drink. They may be expressing a need to toilet or indicating a toileting accident. Children may not have the internal awareness to fully understand what they want. They may use the behavior because they feel an emotion associated with the activity or the event, or they may not know what they want—just that they are frustrated, unhappy, or disappointed. What is their behavior trying to communicate? Is it about the activity that they are doing, or an activity they would rather do instead of the demand you are placing on them?

How the child communicates is as important as what the child is trying to communicate. Is the way the child communicates appropriate? In both Michael and Gabriel's case neither used appropriate communication strategies to get their needs met. Michael needed to request to use the computer, and had he had permission, the urgency of getting to the computer would have been eliminated. Gabriel would quickly have been granted permission to go to the bathroom, had he been able to communicate his need.

Obsessive and compulsive tendencies often result in the child trying to repetitively obtain an object, use a behavior, or repeat a thought. According to LaGrossa (2003), statistics reveal that one in fifty adults in the United States has obsessive-compulsive disorder (OCD). Furthermore, LaGrossa quotes the 1980's National Institute for Mental Health's declaration that OCD affects more than two percent of the population. According to Corboy, in LaGrossa (2003), OCD has a neurological, inheritable, and learned basis. He believes there is an overlap between sensory integrative difficulties and OCD in physiological and sensory respects; OCD, however, is also a cognitive process involving repetitive thoughts. Children and adults with pervasive developmental disorders (PDD) or autism spectrum disorder (ASD) often display the stereotypical behaviors of rigidity and compulsiveness that closely resemble OCD.

An obsession is an internally driven fixation in which the child has a compulsion or preoccupation with a specific toy, activity, or sequence for completing an activity. Examples include seeking out numbers and letters from any environment and arranging them in order, tapping puzzle pieces three times before putting them in, spinning small toys, lining up objects in a row, or stacking them methodically. An uncontrollable need to have a specific toy or activity is another form of obsession, such as letters, numbers, trains, trucks or small sticks. If the child sees them, he or she must have them (Murray-Slutsky and Paris 2000). Objects of obsession are strong primary reinforcers: engaging with the object reinforces itself (Charlop and Haymes 1996).

A child may attempt to obtain a familiar task, activity, or event while resisting the transition to new ones. We know that some children with sensory-related disorders and motor planning difficulties may prefer familiar activities to novel tasks that place increased demands upon them. Other children prefer repetitive activities. It is difficult for them to change an activity, especially to one that is new and unfamiliar. These children will often resist changes from a preferred activity to another.

Just as transition from one task to another is difficult, so is transition from one environment to another. Many children, such as those with autism, may not register what is considered the salient part of the task and may focus on something extraneous. They will often register and enjoy the sensory experience associated with an activity and do not want to terminate it. It is important to identify what aspect of the activity or environment the child is trying to communicate about and perpetuate so that you can plan an intervention to make transitions and new tasks easier.

Obtain

Basic Intervention Principles—Need, Want, Object, or Activity

Obtaining Behaviors

Social Communication — Need, Want, Object, or Activity

Identify what is being communicated. What does the child want or need?

Identify whether the method of communication is acceptable.

- If acceptable, no intervention is necessary.

- If unacceptable, does the child know what he needs or wants? Is he capable of knowing?

If No:

- Anticipate the child's needs.

- Control the environment to make sure the child's needs and wants are met.

- Teach coping skills. Let the child know you are working with him and trying to figure out his needs.

- Teach basic communication strategies. Use picture systems or picture-based computer strategies.

If Yes:

- Establish communication.

- Implement a communication system.

- Be consistent—implement the communication system in all environments.

Identify whether you can give the child the object or activity if he communicates or attempts to communicate correctly.

- If yes, prompt or facilitate communication, then give him what he asked for.

- If no, you cannot give him the activity:

  - Is it something he can earn as a reward?

  - If he becomes angry at not getting the activity, remove it from sight or distract him from the idea or topic and continue with the desired task. Do not attend to angry behavior. Prompt him through the task as needed and praise on-task behavior.

If the child resists the transition to a new activity, insisting on obtaining/maintaining a preferred activity, then:

- Physically transition the child to the new activity.

- Engage the child in the new activity; assist or prompt the child as needed.

- Decrease the amount of assistance or prompts as the child begins to engage.

When working with objects of obsession:

- Whenever possible, use the object as a primary reinforcer for on-task behavior.

- Establish specific criteria the child needs to accomplish in order to obtain the object.

- Reward him with the object for three to five seconds, then remove it and continue with the activity.

When the object is interfering with the activity at hand, is not in the child's best interest, or always presents a problem, you may:

- Set up the environment to make sure the object is NOT available. This is the easiest strategy and avoids a battle.

- Remove the object from the child and from his sight.

  - Do it quickly.

  - Do not rationalize what you did, as this only increases anxiety and provides negative attention.

  - Do not attend to the obsessive behavior.

  - Continue with the desired task.

  - Prompt the child through the transition (see chapter 8, Behavioral Intervention Techniques).

Avoidance or Escape Behaviors
Communication

Children may display challenging behaviors in a conscious effort to avoid situations or activities, or in an unconscious attempt to escape from uncomfortable or unpleasant feelings. Avoidance of tasks, attention, or events falls under the general category of communication. Problematic or challenging behaviors occur when a child displays avoidance or escape behaviors rather than communicating. It is not uncommon for children not to know their needs, wants, and fears, or to be able to relate how they feel to their

"Avoidance" or "Escape" Behaviors

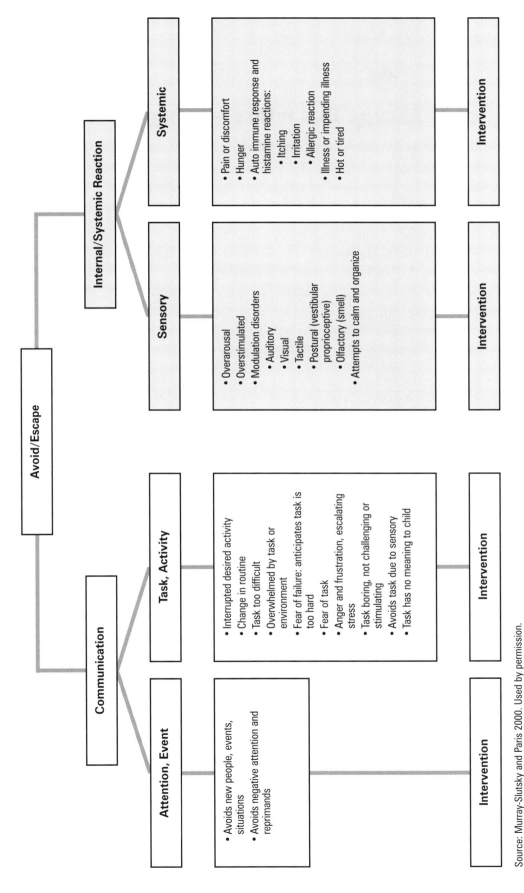

Avoid

Source: Murray-Slutsky and Paris 2000. Used by permission.

Figure 6.2   Analyzing avoidance or escape behaviors—focus on nonsensory communication behaviors

behaviors. Communication strategies become critical to increase these children's insights into their behaviors, provide constructive avenues for communication, and alleviate the underlying problems. By identifying the need that the child is trying to meet, we can develop an effective intervention plan.

Avoidance or Escape Behaviors—Communication

Behaviors to Avoid Attention, People, and Events

Children may avoid situations and activities that are new, including the attention of new as well as familiar people, and new social situations or events. A child who has difficulty functioning, for whatever reason, will attempt to control other people and situations to prevent the stress of new challenges. These children find safety and comfort in routine. In new situations a child can neither control the events that occur, nor assure that he can function effectively, thereby viewing new situations as stressful. It is a natural response to avoid situations that are viewed as stressful.

Avoidance of new activities or events occurs for many different reasons. Children with motor-planning difficulties cannot function if the activities they can perform are altered. New situations threaten their ability to function. Children with defensiveness, modulation difficulties, and other sensory integrative dysfunctions may find new situations difficult when they cannot control or predict the noise levels, when they might be touched or bumped, or the activities that might occur. They may feel especially awkward in social situations. They may have difficulty grasping the whole picture or lack knowledge of the basic or more advanced social skills needed for new situations. They may focus on what appear to be irrelevant aspects of the environment or have difficulty reading implied meaning, subtle innuendo, nonverbal communication, and gestures associated with social situations. They may have difficulty registering changes and initiating actions. They may not register a new person who walked in. If they register the person, they may not know, nor be able to, initiate the appropriate response or greeting.

Children with autism have additional concerns. They often avoid eye contact or ignore even a parent, grandparent, or teacher at times. New people pose a particular threat because they have no idea what demands the new person will make. The social and communication impairments of autism hinder their ability to understand and participate in the verbal exchanges and gestures associated with social situations. Avoidance of eye contact, physical contact, and general interaction can occur for many sensory and nonsensory reasons: voice qualities, pitch, a perfume, the anticipated demands that the person may make, or simply because the child does not want to be bothered.

Basic Intervention Principles—Attention, People, and Events

Avoidance or Escape Behaviors
Communication—Avoiding Attention, People, and Events

The goal is to help the child learn to cope with new situations by teaching exactly what to expect, how to respond appropriately, and to assure that the child has the skills needed to function within new environments. This will lessen the stress and anxiety associated with new places, events, or people, and help him feel more confident.

Establish a method for the child to communicate with you. If the child can attempt to express what he does not like, use an appropriate greeting, or request a small change in the situation, he will not have the need to resort to behaviors.

- Determine what communication method the child understands and will be implemented:

  - Object reference system: The use of objects to represent items or scheduled activities

  - Picture system

  - Signs/gestures

  - Words

Always give structured, positive reinforcement anytime the child is actively engaged in activities or events, or with people he would normally avoid.

Teach the child exactly what he can expect when he attends to, or engages in, the new activity, event, or meets the new person/people.

- Use social stories to familiarize him with the sequence of events that he needs to follow. Social stories are specific short stories designed to be read with the child, once a day initially, to familiarize him with new experiences. Gray (1994) has several social story books available to cover topics including home, community, social and school activities, as well as how to write your own social story (www.thegraycenter.org).

- Familiarize the child with all aspects of the new situation.

- Teach basic social routines. Teach this as part of social stories and within the context of daily activities. Practice in every environment until it is automatic. They include:

  - Look at people when they talk to you.

  - Say hello, goodbye, or wave goodbye when leaving.

  - Respond when another person talks to you.

  - Practice and work on language, pragmatics and social skills to include:

    - Social expectations in different situations (e.g., in class you don't talk, you raise your hand; at recess and in the cafeteria you may talk).

    - Understanding what has been said.

    - Expressing himself accurately, fluently, and appropriately. Give feedback or responses that reinforce his efforts.

    - Understanding semantics, or the context of words, and how they can alter the meaning. For example, "You are next," "You will be last," or "No, in one minute."

    - Matching voice to message—Altering tone of voice to not sound angry, mean, sarcastic, or whining.

    - Getting attention correctly, initiating and maintaining a conversation, listening, adjusting a conversation based on the listener, expressing feelings, stating opinions.

    - Verbal and nonverbal communication.

Avoid

- Practice related activities and responses to make sure the child will feel comfortable with the new activity.

- Make sure the child has the skills needed to do the new activity or participate in the new event.

- Prompt desired behaviors.

- Reward desired behaviors with a primary or secondary reinforcer.

Stephanie, a five-year-old child diagnosed with pervasive developmental delay, has a difficult time with new situations. In these circumstances, she often displays challenging behaviors that include throwing herself on the floor, screaming or making loud noises, banging her head, and lunging or scratching at people nearby.

Stephanie was scheduled to participate in therapeutic horseback riding. Her teachers, parents, behavioralists, and therapists worked together to help her make an easy transition to the new experience of horseback riding. Many activities in the classroom, home, and therapy revolved around horses. Pictures of horses were cut out and posted on the chalkboard and walls at home and school. A social story was developed about a girl who went horseback riding. It described the steps involved in the entire process, from climbing the mounting block and riding the horse, to the people who would be there to assist her, to getting off the horse. The story was read every day at school and at home. There were also discussions about what horses eat, where they live, the texture of their hair, and how big they are. Hay was brought in to the therapy session so Stephanie could connect the sight, smell, and the feel of the hay with the horse. Riding the horse was discussed and Stephanie practiced wearing a helmet and sitting in a saddle attached to a peanut ball. She associated the bouncing (which she enjoyed) with the saddle and the word *horse*. She practiced saying *horse*, making the sounds that signal the horse to move, and learning a song about a horse.

On the first day she rode a horse, all discussions centered on horses and riding, with emphasis on *today*. Stephanie carried a picture of a horse with her while she was being driven to the stables. She made the transition easily, with excitement and enthusiasm. She was guided and prompted up the mounting block and up onto the horse, and she helped to put on her riding helmet. The horse started to move and she quickly associated the movement with the horse. Stephanie knew what to expect and how to respond. There was no anxiety, stress, or fear of the unknown—only pleasure and excitement.

Source: Murray-Slutsky and Paris 2000. Used by permission.

Avoidance or Escape Behaviors
Communication
Behaviors to Avoid Task, Object, or Activity

Children avoid tasks for many reasons. The primary reason is that they possess neither the skills needed to complete a task successfully nor the ability to communicate this effectively. It is important to realize that, while the adult may believe the child is capable of functioning, the child may not believe that he possesses the skills and will act accordingly. The child's fear, frustration, and stress often are expressed in task avoidance and escape behaviors that can quickly develop into fleeing the area, distractibility and avoidance strategies, or self-abusive or aggressive behaviors as the child's frustration mounts.

We must analyze the task, the environment, and the child's skills and emotional responses in order to determine the primary cause for the child's behavior. Then, we must modify the environment, grade the task, and help the child succeed while convincing the child that he is indeed capable.

The *task analysis* involves breaking the activity into its component parts:

- What physical skills does the task require?

- Is it an exciting, boring, or unstimulating task?

- Is there sensory feedback associated with the task? What is it? How much?

- Is it a new task that the child has never seen or attempted, or an activity that is out of his routine?

- Is it simple or complex?

- Is the presentation overwhelming or are the component parts clearly visible?

Avoid

The *skills analysis* involves analyzing the child's functional skills:

- Does the child actually possess the skills needed to complete the task at the level of independence in which it is being presented?

  - Does he possess all of the skills needed or only some of them?

  - Can he do the skill with several different people and in different contexts? Some children cannot generalize skills to perform around other people or in different environments.

- Does he have the sensory-motor awareness to complete the task?

- Is his sensory system over- or undersensitive? In which systems?

- Is the task developmentally- or age-appropriate for the child? Is it too childish or too high level for him?

The *emotional analysis* involves analyzing how and why the child emotionally responds to the task:

- Is the child reacting emotionally with fight, flight, or fright? (Is there an autonomic nervous system (ANS) response with increased heart rate, dilated pupils, and flushing of the skin? If the child has an ANS reaction, and it is ignored (you continue to push the child), the child may react with aggression.)

  - Aggression turned inward may result in forms of self-abuse such as biting or head banging.

  - Aggression turned outward may result in you being bitten, slapped, or pinched.

- Is the response due to decreased self-confidence or self-esteem?

- Is the response rooted in fear? The child may fear the task because:

  - He feels it is beyond his capabilities.

  - He fears failure.

  - He lacks confidence and self-esteem.

- Does the response occur:

  - With an identifiable need or want?

  - When he is excited, mad, or distressed?

- ▪ When he is angry or frustrated?

- ▪ When he needs a break or help with the task?

- ■ Is the child responding emotionally out of boredom?

- ■ Is the child responding to the sensory component of the task? This will often occur in the child with hyperresponsiveness or defensiveness within a particular system.

After analyzing the task, the child's skills and his emotional response, you should have a grasp on the underlying problem. These frequently fall into one of the following categories:

- ■ The task is too difficult.

- ■ The task or activity has no meaning or purpose to the child.

- ■ The task is boring, unstimulating, or not challenging.

- ■ The task is overwhelming.

- ■ The task is a change in routine and the child is having difficulty adjusting.

- ■ The child dislikes the task.

- ■ The child lacks self-confidence.

- ■ The child fears the task.

- ■ The child is reacting to a sensory component of the task.

Children avoid tasks that they perceive as boring, unstimulating, and having no purpose or challenge. Koomar and Bundy (2002) identified the responsibility of the therapy profession to find the just-right challenge, in which the child is motivated and invested in the activity. Finding this level requires a comprehensive knowledge of the child's abilities and of what will motivate him. Underestimating the child's capabilities can be equally as deleterious as overestimating them. Children often will rise to the occasion when people know their capabilities, place expectations slightly above that point, and simultaneously project to them that they believe in their capabilities and will provide support and encouragement.

Children with decreased sensory awareness often find activities meaningless and unstimulating. They require enhanced sensory experiences during the activity for them to understand how to use their arms, legs, hands, and feet to accomplish the task and to gain pleasure from participating in it.

A task may also be overstimulating for the child. Tasks presented in an unstructured, disorganized, ungraded fashion can result in the child either shutting down or exhibiting avoidance or escape behaviors. This can occur even though the task is well within the child's capabilities. The presentation of a task and the environment in which the task is performed can account for a child's varying functional levels with different adults.

Another cause of task avoidance involves a defensiveness or aversion to the sensory components within the task. Overresponsive, defensive children often demonstrate avoidance behaviors because of smells or textures involved in the task. To address these issues a therapist would treat the underlying cause; the teacher or parent might substitute the substances used within the activity to gain compliance.

Lastly, because change is difficult for many children, transitions between activities and interruptions in their desired activity can lead to frustration and stress and result in behaviors that are less than optimal. The task is a change in routine and the child is having difficulty adjusting. We must be careful to prepare children either verbally or visually that a change will occur. Assist them through the transition, and engage them in the next activity. Avoid downtime if at all possible.

Basic Intervention Principles—Task, Object, or Activity

Avoidance or Escape Behaviors
Communication — Task, Object, or Activity Avoidance

To extinguish the need for behaviors as a communication strategy a child must have an alternative method by which to communicate. This may involve gestures, signs, pictures, or some other form of augmentative communication. Then, the child needs to be taught what he wants or what he is reacting to, and how to communicate that in an acceptable manner. Primary or secondary reinforcers may be needed to reinforce the new methods of communication while extinguishing the undesired behavior.

Once the child has learned the new communication technique, begin building in delayed gratification and fading out the use of primary reinforcers. Teach the child self-regulation techniques so that he does not get frustrated and lose control over his behaviors when delayed gratification is called for. Remember that the child must be successful in his attempts at communication lest he revert to old behaviors or invent new strategies.

Intervene before the behavior occurs; design a program to eliminate the need for the behavior, and then to eliminate the behavior itself.

Establish a method for the child to communicate with you.

Always give structured, positive reinforcement anytime the child is actively engaged in activities and events.

Avoidance of task, object, or event
- Identify the aspect of the task or activity the child is avoiding and determine the reason for task avoidance.
  - Perform a task analysis.
  - Perform a skills analysis.
  - Analyze the child's emotional response.

The task that is too difficult
The task may be beyond the child's capability or the child may actually possess the skills, but emotionally believes the task is too difficult. When the task is beyond the child's capability you may:
- Modify the task; making it easier, thereby guaranteeing the child can successfully complete it.
  - Match the task to the child's functional level. It will promote independence and decrease the likelihood of challenging behaviors.
  - Provide emotional support and encouragement.
  - Provide positive reinforcement and praise for accomplishing the task.
  - Gradually increase the level of difficulty as the child's skills increase.
  - Improve the underlying skill that resulted in the task being too difficult.

- Keep the task at the current level but provide assistance to the child.

  - Provide physical, verbal, or visual assistance to the aspect of the task that is too difficult so he can successfully complete the task. See chapter 8, Behavioral Intervention Techniques.

  - Provide emotional support, giving positive feedback and encouragement.

  - Improve skills needed to perform the task successfully.

Avoid

The child possesses the skills needed for the task, but does not believe he possesses them. This is usually due to lack of self confidence, self esteem, or lack of awareness or exposure to successfully complete the task.

- Positively reinforce the child's skills as you gradually increase independence in task completion.

- Keep the task at the current level of difficulty while providing support and encouragement.

- Delayed reinforcement and prompting (see chapter 8, Behavioral Intervention Techniques) are effective in increasing a child's confidence and independence without triggering frustration.

- Give the child additional exposure to the task, have him repeat it several times in different settings.

- Be careful not to verbalize and rationalize as an attempt to coax the child through the task, as it may provide negative attention and reinforcement.

- Positively reinforce him as he constructively works on the task and again at task completion with attention and confirmation that you knew he could do it.

When a child avoids activities because he perceives them as too difficult:

- Do not allow the child to escape the activity.

- Reward any effort at performance of task.

Task is viewed as boring, not stimulating, not challenging, or overwhelming

The task is below the child's skill level, or is too easy for him. This often results in inattention and complaints that the activity is boring or unstimulating.

- Modify the task to increase the challenge as appropriate.

The task may not have inherent sensory feedback necessary to engage the child.

- Enhance the sensory feedback in the task. Analyze what type of sensory feedback the child needs in order to engage in the activity (see Table 10.1 to alter arousal levels through therapeutic use of self and environmental factors, and appendix A for intervention for underresponsiveness). For example:

  - An underaroused child may need instructions presented in an enthusiastic manner with a strong voice volume.

  - A child undersensitive to touch may have difficulty maneuvering a pencil in his hand and may respond better with enhanced sensory feedback: a weighted pencil, sandpaper under the writing surface, or writing on an inclined surface.

The task or activity lacks meaning or purpose to the child.

- Increase sensory registration.

- Attach meaning to the activity.

- Connect the idea of the task to the end product.

- Increase sensory feedback (refer to "the task may not have inherent sensory feedback" above).

- Many activities must be completed that have no meaning to the child (learning the alphabet, writing). To increase compliance, build in reinforcers. See chapter 8, Behavioral Intervention Techniques.

Downtime within and between activities can result in boredom and task avoidance from the child.

- Be prepared and organized. Look at ways to modify the environment to increase your efficiency.

- Decrease downtime between activities.

Task is not interesting.

- Increase enthusiasm about the activity. Increase your animation.

- Increase the child's investment in the activity.

- Build rewards and reinforcers into the activity.

The task is viewed as overwhelming, and may be disorganized and unstructured.

- Analyze the task and the environment for both the amount of structure and stimulation provided.

- Modify the environment to decrease over stimulation. Increase structure and boundaries, prevent shut down, and increase interest. (See chapter 7, Environmental Intervention Techniques.)

- Grade the task; break it into its component parts. Present one item at a time.

- Avoid irrelevant or distracting instructions (i.e., avoid too many words).

Child dislikes the task.

- Set a low minimum performance level.

- Convey that performance level visually to the child.

- Immediately reward and encourage on-task behavior. Reward task completion. Work toward delayed gratification (see chapter 8, Behavioral Intervention Techniques).

Avoidance triggered by transitions; child has difficulty with change

- Establish systems and routines.

- Prepare the child visually and verbally prior to the transition.

- Have the next activity organized and structured.

- Assist in moving the child through the transition and engaging in the next activity without waiting time.

Avoidance due to a lack of self-confidence

- Provide encouragement and emotional support as needed.

- Offer assistance or prompts to complete the task. Reward on-task behavior and task completion. Fade prompts as soon as possible.

- Reward the child's efforts immediately and consistently. Draw attention to, and reinforce, task completion to increase self-confidence.

- Gradually fade attention to intermittent reinforcement (every third to fourth time) as his success increases.

- Address or respond to the child's emotional responses (anger, frustration, happiness, and need for help).

Avoidance due to fear of the task or sensory components

- If the fear is rational (has a definite cause or reason) address the underlying cause. For example:

  - If the child lacks postural control and balance because of vestibular and proprioceptive difficulties, he may avoid moveable equipment or elevated surfaces. In such cases the therapist must address any postural insecurity and build in the necessary motor control.

  - If the child avoids the task because of an underresponsiveness to sensory input, the adult must find a way to enhance the sensory component.

  - Finally, if the avoidance stems from a defensiveness, deep-proprioceptive activities must be added to regulate the child's overresponsiveness to the sensory components of the task.

- If the fear appears irrational or does not appear to have an objective cause, then treat the underlying sensory processing issues (refer to sensory based avoidance behaviors).

  - Be supportive and positive in the child's efforts.

Environmental Intervention Techniques

7

Many behaviors can be extinguished or avoided simply by engineering an environment that makes problem behaviors less apt to occur. The primary goal of intervention is to create an environment for the child in which he does not need to use the behaviors. Whether the underlying cause is sensory or behavioral, environmental considerations are of great importance. Environmental considerations include not only the physical, structural environment, but also such things as background noise, lighting, and visual clutter, as well as people within the child's environment and task presentation.

Engineering the Environment

Children with sensory integrative and behavioral disorders have difficulty organizing themselves, selecting what is appropriate to attend to and what is extraneous to the task at hand. By engineering the physical setting to decrease clutter, you can promote attention to salient components within both the physical setting and a given activity.

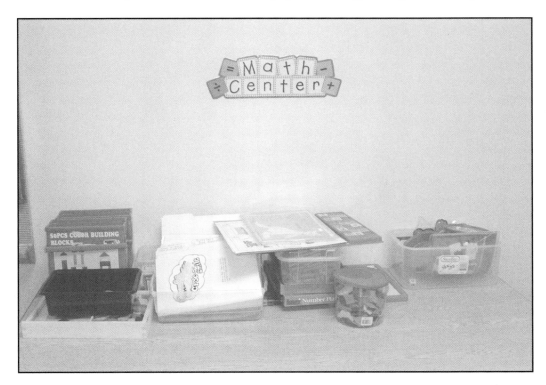

Delineate workspace visually.

Small or Subdivided Room

Behaviors are much more likely to occur in a large, open room. Large spaces have no inherent boundaries to help a child sustain a sense of organization and control. A child who has difficulty with organization and staying on task will have even greater difficulty in a large, unstructured area, such as a large, open classroom, cafeteria, gymnasium, grocery store, or library. Large spaces must be visually separated and work areas defined. Large spaces may be visually structured into smaller spaces by subdividing the room, using furniture placement, or delineating workspaces visually.

Children may not inherently understand the structure that exists within large, open spaces. They may panic, become overwhelmed with fear, or run. Other children may simply lose their ability to focus and organize themselves. Impulsivity, hyperactivity, distractibility, and unbridled acting out may be their reactions to the environment. Teaching the child to understand the structure, to know where he needs to go, to see the smaller parts that make up the whole, and to focus only on the salient aspects within the environment are important. In the grocery store, placing a young child in the cart or teaching an older child to push the cart while simultaneously teaching him the system that exists within each row will help them understand boundaries and how to function.

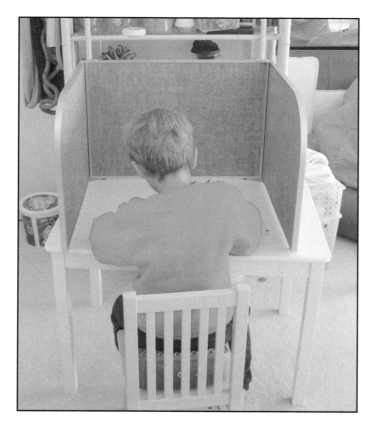

Study-Rite Carrels reduce distractions and help students concentrate while providing a personal work environment.

In school, all that the young child may need is a carpet on which to sit, thereby defining the space that he must occupy during circle time. A work desk at the front of a classroom or facing a wall or a cubicle in which to work can also help the child define his space. Colored tape used to mark lines on the floor can separate large areas and help a child move from one class to another or keep in line behind classmates. Classrooms can be arranged to make specific areas for different tasks, such as reading, deskwork, or circle time. Partitions or furniture can define the separate areas. Look at ways to subdivide cafeterias and decrease the noise level through using partitions or carpet. When this can't be done, position the child at a table in a quieter corner. Have the child face a wall, or have his back to everyone coming in. In large open environments, the child must learn to define the boundaries (the structure that exists within chaos) and the expectations for behavior in order to function.

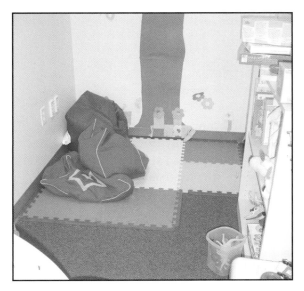 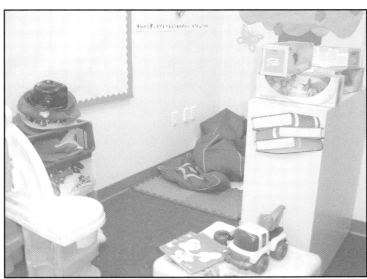

Within a large room, use partitions or carpeting to create quiet areas and calming centers.

Noise and Sound Levels

Auditory stimulation (high noise level) has been identified as a catalyst in a child with hyperresponsiveness or defensiveness, self-regulatory, and auditory processing issues. It is also frequently cited as an area of difficulty for children with autism. Auditory stimulation within the environment can quickly escalate a child's level of arousal and stress, negatively affecting his ability to register and process information, and therefore, function. However, overarousal may not be the only problem encountered. If the child's auditory skills are weak, the stimulation may negatively affect the child's auditory processing or create auditory overload.

Simply put, auditory processing is what the brain does with what the ear hears (Katz and Wilde 1994). Auditory processing is responsible for localizing, lateralizing, and discriminating sounds. It contributes to auditory attention, discrimination, and recognition. Most children with auditory processing problems have normal intelligence and normal hearing sensitivity (Florida Department of Education 2001), but in order to learn, a child must be able to attend to, listen to, and separate important speech from all other noises at school and home. When auditory skills are weak, the child may experience auditory overload.

Auditory overload may be caused by:

- Fast rate of speaking
- Rapid presentation of new information

- Speech that is too complex or that sounds the same (phonetically similar)

- Reduced context: Talking without visual or situational support to make meaning of what is said

- Increased length of decontextualized material: Too much talking without visual or situational support to make meaning of what is said

- Decreased word familiarity

- Increased specificity of expected response: Demanding a response in a short time

- Increased task uncertainty: Open tasks without structure

- Poor listening conditions: Background noises, distance from speaker, and reverberation

Auditory processing involves hearing what is said, decoding what is said, and remembering what is said long enough to comply with what is asked. It is important to monitor the child's reaction to you personally. You may need to aid the child by modulating your own voice and altering the pitch, the number of words you use, and the rate at which you speak. It may be necessary to allow for increased processing times and to lessen the amount of verbal instruction so the child can process what you want.

Table 7.1
Checklist of Strategies to Reduce Distractions

(A) auditory   (V) visual   (O) organizational   (OS) other sensory

Ceiling considerations	
Acoustic ceiling tiles	A
Ceiling height should be less than 12 feet high	A
Flooring	
Rubberized or resilient tile	A
Carpeting installed over padding	A
Carpeting extends over the bottom of the wall	A
Hallways and adjoining areas are carpeted	A
Area rugs	A
Wall coverings	
Cork bulletin boards	A
Felt or flannel boards	A
Acoustical or fabric covered wall	A
Window coverings	A
Artwork on walls	A

(*continued*)

Table 7.1 Checklist of Strategies to Reduce Distractions (*Continued*)

Wall coverings (continued)

Type and amount of pictures hung on wall or from ceilings is kept to a minimum	V
Items are not being blown by the wind or air-conditioning	V

Window covering

Drapes	A
Artwork on windows	A

Doors and doorways

Solid core doors	A
Noise-lock seal, felt doorway lining	A
Draft guard or doors covered	A

Furniture

Staggered desks	A
Desk and chair leg bottoms padded or covered	A
Bulletin boards, bookcases, file cabinets placed to break up space	A,V
Study carrels	A, V

Light fixtures

Housing for fluorescent light should be above acoustical tile in ceiling	A
Ballasts must be changed on a regular basis	A

Instructional methods

Instruction occurs away from noise sources: heating, air-conditioning vents	A
Background noise kept to a minimum	A
Task presentation is organized with extraneous supplies and work out of sight	O,V
Clean up after each project	O,V
Tasks are presented in manageable parts	O,V
Placement of learning activity is appropriate from the child's perspective	O,V

Other sensory distractions

Distracting smells are avoided whenever possible	OS
Temperature of room is maintained at a comfortable level	OS

Reducing noise and reverberation (or echo) helps everyone function in a stress-free environment. In schools, reducing classroom noise and reverberation makes listening, learning, and teaching more pleasant and improves morale and motivation.

Acoustical ceiling tiles are the most effective way of absorbing distorted middle- and high-frequency noise and improving speech-perception ability. Ceiling heights less than twelve feet are optimal for the listening environment.

Carpeting installed over a pad is the most effective and efficient acoustical modification for absorbing excessive reverberation of high-frequency consonant sounds and dampening noise from students and movement of furniture. Noise is further reduced if carpet is extended onto the bottom portion of the wall. Carpeting hallways next to classrooms helps to reduce external noise. Reflective floor surfaces, such as tile, reflect sound. Rubberized or resilient tile absorbs more noise than a flat, reflective surface. Area rugs or carpets may also decrease noise levels.

Windows, walls, chalkboards, and doors are highly reflective. Draperies, blinds, and shades provide acoustical treatment for windows. Cloth draperies with rubberized backing are most effective in reducing noise and reverberation. If installing drapes is not possible, applying student artwork and charts to the windows provides some acoustical modifications. Cork bulletin boards, felt or flannel boards, and walls covered in acoustical tile or fabric are useful in reducing noise and reverberation. A solid-core door provides better acoustic capabilities than a hollow-core door. Doors should fit well in the doorway to help lessen noise from outside or adjacent areas. A noise-lock seal can be installed or a felt lining added around a doorway to lessen external sound.

The human body absorbs sound. When desks are staggered, sound will not travel directly and reflect off the walls. Putting felt caps or tennis balls on chair and table legs helps reduce noise in uncarpeted areas. Mobile bulletin boards and bookcases placed at angles with the walls can decrease reverberation in the classroom and may also be useful in partially blocking noise from computers, the bathroom, or learning center areas. Study carrels can serve as room dividers and can also break up noise. They can also be lined with acoustical tiles to reduce equipment noise.

Some fluorescent lights emit a constant noise. The hum can be partially eliminated if the ballasts are changed on a regular basis. If lighting is housed above the acoustical tile ceiling, the noise level will be lessened.

Arranging the classroom so that instruction occurs away from the noise source is recommended. If the classroom has an external heating, ventilation and air-conditioning system, as is the case with most portable units, instruction should occur away from the vents.

Creating an atmosphere that is calm and organized and facilitates learning can be aided with the careful selection of music. Classical music, such as Mozart or Baroque, or music with strong rhythmic components played at low volumes can have a calming and relaxing impact on children with heightened arousal levels, oversensitivity, or defensiveness. Environmental factors can enhance the learning environment and set a child up for good behavior (Florida Department of Education 2001).

Whether the environment is too stimulating or noisy depends on the individual child's response, not on how others perceive it. Similarly, not all calming strategies work for all children, and recommended strategies must be assessed based upon the response of each child.

Visual Distractions

Most children are easily distracted by visuals (people and objects) in their environment, especially those children with sensory integrative dysfunctions. Children with poor internal organization and higher sensory thresholds (hypersensitive) will have difficulty knowing what to focus on within the environment. These children may have difficulty processing information coming in from more than one sense (multisensory processing), and either attend to everything indiscriminately, or overwhelm and shut down.

Therefore, it is important to consider the type and amount of pictures hung on the wall and items dangling from the ceiling or being blown by the wind, a fan, or an air-conditioner. While many of these objects are intended to brighten up a room, a child may find them distracting, or worse, disorganizing to the point of making the child unable to continue to attend or participate.

Monitor the area you live and work in, assessing it for undue clutter, disorganization, or visual distractions. Make sure large pieces of equipment or unused supplies are neatly stored out of sight. If possible, use partitions to visually block off storage areas.

Table 7.2
Strategies and Systems to Increase Performance

Small rooms	■ Use small, enclosed rooms or subdivide larger rooms with portable partitions or bookcases.
Defined boundaries	■ Set boundaries for expectations and behaviors.
Noise levels	■ Keep noise levels and reverberation to a minimum.
Visual distractions	■ Eliminate extraneous distractions on the walls. Post only pertinent information.
Task presentation	■ Break tasks into manageable parts.
	■ Minimize down time within sessions and during transitions.
	■ Gather needed supplies in advance. Keep them close-by but out of sight until needed.
	■ Take out only the supplies needed at the time.
	■ Put away all equipment when finished with a task.
	■ When appropriate, make cleanup a part of the activity.
	■ If it is inappropriate to spend time on cleanup, move used supplies out of the child's view, proceed to the next activity, and put them away later.
Sensory distractions	■ Modifications may be required based on the child's primary need. Consider smells, number and proximity of other children, temperature, noise, and visual distractions.
Emotional environment	■ Provide a nurturing, positive, and supportive environment.
Strategies and systems	■ Follow a plan. Use schedules, post activities, or use picture schedules. Minimize down time. Be prepared.
	■ Make transitions seamless.
	■ Give advance notice of transitions.
	■ Prepare the child for the change; give concrete reminders of time remaining or amount of work left before the transition.
	■ Use a preferred item to distract the child through the transition. Reinforce the child for focusing on the new task.
	■ Begin each session with the same first activity.
	■ Give choices and a degree of control. Give concrete choices or help the child organize an acceptable choice.

(continued)

Table 7.2 Strategies and Systems to Increase Performance (*Continued*)

Strategies and systems (continued)	■ Set the rules. Visually display rules. Review them before the activity.
	■ Give instructions concisely. Eliminate extraneous verbalizations.
	■ Utilize behavioral momentum. Build a momentum of positive "yes" answers, then present a less-preferred task.
Concise instructions	■ Limit extraneous verbalizations.
	■ Monitor your instructions; be brief and concise.
	■ Do not ask whether a child wants to do something unless you are prepared to let him or her decline.
	■ Keep verbalizations specific to the task, especially when a child is just learning words.
	■ Use gestures with verbal instructions to help increase comprehension.
	■ If necessary, limit instructions to one or two words.
Defined rules	■ Teach rules that help children succeed.
	■ Specify rules clearly and concisely.
	■ Be sure the child understands the rules and consequences, if any.
	■ Help the child link the action with the consequence.
	■ Enforce rules consistently.
	■ Post the rules.
	■ Review the rules with the children before they need to use them.
Positive behavioral momentum	■ Encourage "yes" answers and minimize negative responses.
	■ Ask the child to comply with several easy tasks, reward the efforts, and praise the child.
	■ After building a momentum of positive responses, present the less-preferred task, and praise and reinforce all efforts.
Interesting activities	■ Create tasks that are interesting, motivating, and challenging because they keep children engrossed.
Quantifiable tasks	■ Let the child know the end point of tasks.
	■ Specify how many items are to be completed.
	■ Break tasks into component parts that appear manageable to the child.

Source: Murray-Slutsky and Paris 2000. Used by permission.

Task Presentation

Task presentation involves organizing the activity in advance. Gather specific supplies and equipment and have them ready but out of the child's sight. For the child who has difficulty organizing and sequencing a task or who cannot discern what is important and what is extraneous to the task, it is important to place supplies in a container or box and take out only what is needed at the time. Place items in clear view if you want the child to see and use them. Keep them out of the child's view if you are not yet ready to have the child focus on them.

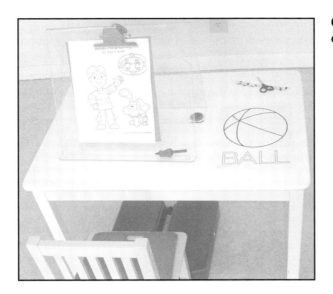

Gather specific supplies and equipment in advance.

Break tasks into parts that appear manageable. Present a limited number of items for the child to complete. If you are asking the child to make a picture by gluing items onto paper, present the items one or two at a time. Behaviors often erupt when a box of glue sticks, markers, and items to be glued are scattered on the desktop. Look at the task from the child's perspective: Is it manageable or is it overwhelming? Worksheets can appear cluttered and overwhelming to a child. Teaching the child to cover up everything but the first line, using a template that covers everything on the page but one question or math problem, and folding the page in half are strategies to help the child break the task into manageable parts. The child who does not know where to begin, cannot see an end to the task, or is inundated by the presentation of a task rapidly becomes overwhelmed and frustrated.

Put away all supplies and equipment as you finish each task. Be aware that you can easily lose control of a child by losing control of the environment. Assist the child to put toys in their containers or in their assigned place. If you cannot dedicate time to cleanup, move all used supplies out of the child's visual field and engage the child in the next activity. Once the child is engrossed in the new activity, you may put away previously used supplies.

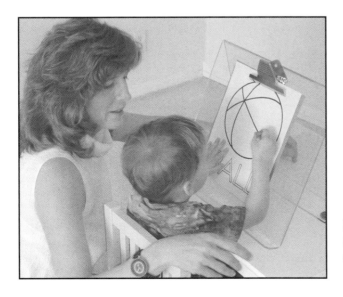

Present a limited number of items for the child to complete.

It is also important to consider whether the placement of the activity is appropriate from the child's perspective. Ask yourself if the child realizes that the activity applies to him. A common example is the shared use of a computer in pre-primary grades. Often two or more children are placed in front of the computer screen and assisted by an adult. When two or more children share a monitor, the child with sensory processing problems may not realize that the monitor is the salient point to the task. He may focus instead on the keyboard or mouse and may not attend to the monitor at all. The monitor must be at desk or table height for the child and placed at a distance of about two feet from the child to capture the child's visual attention.

Other Sensory Distractions

Odors and temperature regulation contribute to sensory distractions for children. Have you ever been working quietly and the smell of popcorn wafted into the room and lingered? Children rapidly become focused on getting popcorn to eat, to the exclusion of whatever else you may be trying to get them to do. Room temperature can also be a distraction. The child who is uncomfortably warm or cold will not be able to concentrate and will become out-of-sorts and disorganized.

Emotional Environment

A positive, nurturing, and supportive environment is one in which all children flourish. Such an environment is not always easy to provide for the child with problematic or challenging behaviors that test your patience. People in the child's environment must be able to see his positive characteristics and look beyond the problem behaviors. Children have an innate ability to sense when people like them and believe in them and their abilities, and they respond positively in an environment of mutual trust and respect. You project a positive emotional environment through your verbal and nonverbal behavior. It is important to seek to understand the individual child, encourage his participation, respond to his needs, and praise or reward him for on-task, desired behaviors. *Catch the child doing something right and reward him, consistently and often!* Make him believe you respect him, trust in his abilities, and like him.

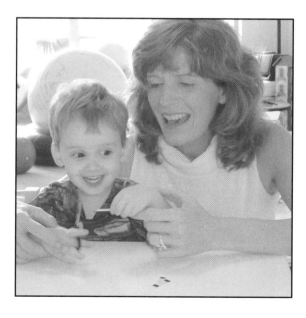

Project a positive, nurturing environment.

Maximize Strategies and Systems

Everyone functions better in environments where they know what to anticipate and what is expected of them. Stress levels increase when the unexpected occurs or when people are not sure of how to perform or react. Desired behavior and compliance increase when you convey to the child what will occur throughout his day and what is expected of him. Problematic or challenging behaviors are provoked when children neither understand nor know what to expect. Here are examples of systems and strategies that work:

Follow a schedule: Have a plan.

Schedules come in many forms: day planners, assignment books, calendars, lists, and the ever-popular refrigerator chart, among others. Teachers often have lists of activities and time schedules written on the board for children to reference. Children with SI dysfunction and organizational difficulties benefit from using a schedule within their daily routine. Schedules may be either visual representations (pictures) or a written list and may include activities for the entire day or week. For some children, knowing the next activity is all that they can cope with. You may present a picture or simply say to the child, "When we finish eating, we will do writing."

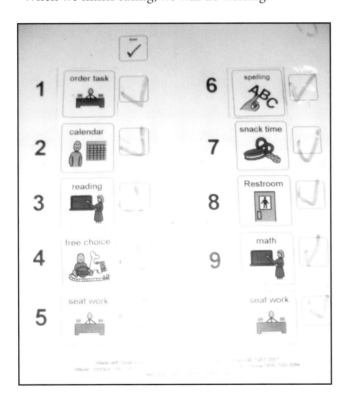

Have a schedule. It may be written or consist of visual representations.

It is important to remember that schedules and time are abstract concepts. They are projections into the future (feedforward) and require an understanding of time and space. Many children are concrete—operating in the present—and have not yet developed the concept of what will happen in the future. When they cannot anticipate the future, it may suffice to verbally explain to them, "First we ___, then we ____." Visual or pictorial schedules are concrete representations of time that can aid the child who cannot read or who has language comprehension or auditory processing difficulties. Understanding time is very difficult for many children to grasp. For example: "In five minutes we will do_____." The Time Timer®, available through therapy equipment vendors, visually depicts time as a red space. The greater the amount of time, the greater the amount of red space. The red space lessens as time goes by. It helps the child visually and internally understand this abstract concept.

Picture schedules are also a helpful way to teach children the sequence of activities throughout the day, helping them understand the concept of the future (feed-forward). Select pictures to depict each activity. Arrange them on a board to show the sequence of activities. After each activity is completed, have the child take the picture off the board or turn it face down on the board to indicate that the activity has ended and it is time to proceed to the next one. To help the child understand the concept of the past or past events (feedback), have the child review the pictures that he has just completed.

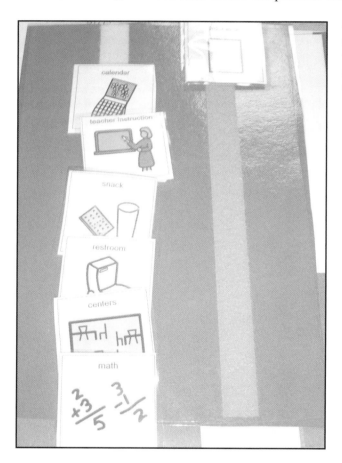

Simple (linear) picture schedules are also helpful to teach the child the sequence of activities and the concept of time.

Minimize downtime.

A child with decreased internal organization and difficulty organizing his behaviors will not be able to organize free time or down time within activities. It is the time many problematic behaviors erupt. Teachers or therapists may unknowingly keep the child waiting as they collect needed supplies, help another child, turn to talk to an adult in the room, or give the child free time as a reward for completing the work, thus innocently setting the environment for the child to misbehave. Children who find themselves with free time frequently do not know what to do, what is expected, or the options to keep themselves busy, productive, and out of trouble. Although parents and teachers expect children to learn to wait, waiting is not an inherently easy task for children. Moments can seem an eternity for children who have self-regulatory problems or SI dysfunction or who do not have the internal control to self-organize. They find waiting exceptionally difficult.

Preparation is the key to minimizing down time. Plan ahead and have what you need readily available. Keep the child engaged and the activities moving to sustain the child's interest. Your goal needs to be to reduce or eliminate down time from the child's schedule. If down time cannot be prevented, keep the child engaged either physically or mentally. A child may need to learn exactly how to organize himself during down time. You may have the child play with a toy or fidget, complete a specific activity, or count from one to ten while you get the necessary items. If you find that the child will not stay still and wait, try having him close his eyes and count backwards from ten to one or from a higher number based upon his skill level. Closing his eyes may help him avoid visual distractions and temptations. Counting backward slows him down slightly, giving you more time to organize. If you cannot use either of these strategies, take the child with you to help get the supplies.

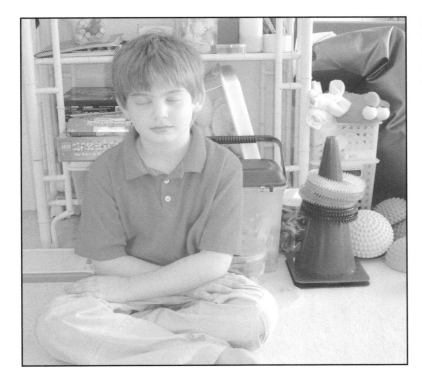

Have the child close his eyes to avoid visual distractions and temptations.

Make transitions as seamless as possible.

Change makes many children anxious. Transitions between activities represent change. They also represent unknown expectations, task demands, and possibly the cessation of a preferred activity. Transitions can trigger anxiety, stress, and behaviors that are difficult to manage. Included here are several techniques that make transitions smoother and less stressful for children, thereby setting the child up for optimal behavior.

Begining with the same first activity or in the same spot within the room each day will decrease the anxiety associated with not knowing what to expect. Establish simple rules the child can follow and make sure the child understands them. At home you may tell the child, "When you wake up in the morning, you will go to the bathroom and then come to breakfast." In the therapy clinic the instruction might be, "When you come in, you will sit here and take your shoes off." In school the child may be told, "Put your things in your cubby and take your seat."

Give advance notice that the activity will soon end and what the next activity will be. Count down the last few repetitions or moments until the change or transition begins, "We have four more, three, two before we change, one, and now we change." Visual strategies often help. Visually place the last four objects the child needs to complete in front of him. If the child needs to complete four worksheets, you may place four small objects in front of him, taking one away every time he completes a page. A picture schedule system may be used to let the child know what the next activity will be. Placing the next activity in clear sight and indicating to the child that this activity will be next is another strategy.

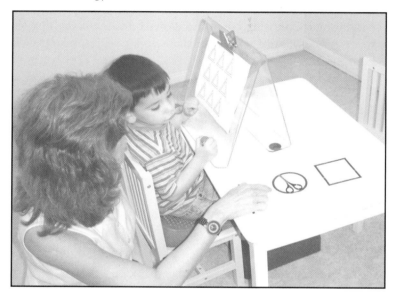

Give advance notice that the activity will soon end and what the next activity will be.

Give the child choices and a degree of control.

Do not set up a power struggle between you and the child. Offer the child a choice of two items or activities. "We must do A and B. Which would you like to do first?" Give the child the choice between two activities that are similar. "You may do this writing page or this one. Which would you like to do?" Avoid asking, "Do you want to __?" unless you are prepared to accept no for an answer.

Be cautious when allowing the child open-ended choices, for example, "I will choose the first activity; then you can choose the second activity." Many children are skillful in avoiding work and distracting you from your goal. They may choose a lengthy activity with no therapeutic or functional value. A child may not consciously be avoiding work but instead may have difficulty organizing and structuring such a request. Your goal may be to help the child learn to structure and organize an open-ended choice. You may teach the child what makes up an acceptable choice, or let the child choose the activity while giving yourself the right to modify it to make it harder. Then work with the child on sequencing and planning the task appropriately.

Allowing the child to choose his reward for work completed correctly is a well-accepted practice. Cipani (1998) describes the use of the Premack principle to increase a child's compliance. The child is allowed access to a preferred event in response to compliance with a request or a task. "You may listen to music, after you write three spelling words" (p. 69).

Set the rules.

Children respond well to guidelines. They learn and abide by simple rules. Rules need to tell the child exactly what the child should be doing. The pitfalls we all fall into are telling the child "Don't _____." When told not to do something, many children lack the knowledge and ability to discern for themselves what they should do. Furthermore, some children only process or remember the last word said. "Don't run," gets interpreted as "run." Get into the habit of making rules positive. Telling a child what not to do (e.g., "Don't run.") reinforces the exact behavior you want to avoid. Whenever possible, rules should be written, visually displayed, and reviewed with the child daily. State the rules specifically and in positive terms. Clearly and succinctly define the exact behavior you want. For example, instead of "No running allowed," you should use the more positive form, "Walk slowly." Make sure that the child understands both the rule and the consequences, if there are any. If the child runs, stop him. Does he understand what he did? Ask him what he was doing. If he doesn't understand, tell him that he was running and ask him what the rule is (i.e., to walk slowly). In either case, immediately and physically take him back and make him walk at an acceptable pace. If he continues to run, tell him he was not walking slowly, repeat the rule, and remove him from the area. Make sure to connect the consequence immediately to the undesired behavior. If there is a delay in the consequence, chances are the child will not associate the consequence with the behavior. Consistency is mandated. If everyone does not enforce rules consistently, the behavior will not be effectively dealt with.

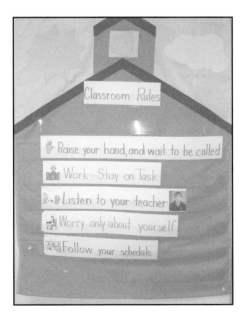

Rules should be written, visually depicted, and reviewed with children daily.

Give instructions concisely.

Children often have difficulty with auditory processing and understanding verbal directions and instructions for a variety of reasons. For most children, the auditory system is not their strongest sense and the meaning conveyed is too abstract for them to fully understand. Often adults use words that children do not comprehend or simply talk too much for the children's abilities. To be understood, give short, concise instructions that may consist of only one or two words. Use gesture or a demonstration with verbal instructions to aid the child's comprehension. Limit your verbalizations to specific tasks or requests, especially if the child is just learning words. Eliminate extraneous questions, such as, "Do you like __?"

If you are repeating directions too many times, try a different strategy. The child may respond better with visual supports, such as a check-off list of things to do, picture system for instructions, gestures or nonverbal instructions, or structured written rules. Stickers or secondary reinforcers may be coupled with these visual supports to provide more incentive.

At Henry's parent-teacher conference the teacher lamented that she had to repeat the directions ten to twelve times for him. His psychologist explained that he obviously had problems following verbal directions. She recommended visual instructions and cues rather than verbal ones. Checking tasks off a written list could help Henry understand and plan the sequence of activities he needs to complete. The teacher would point to the ones that still had to be done and reward him when he completed the entire list without prompting.

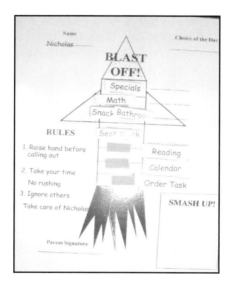

The rocket defines rules specific to each child and the activity schedule provides a reward at the end of the day if the tasks are completed.

Use positive behavioral momentum.

Some children start every task by saying, "No." By engaging in a debate after the child says, "No," you are only encouraging further negative responses. To avoid further negative responses make use of behavioral momentum. *Behavioral momentum* is a strategy that encourages "yes" answers and minimizes negative responses. Start with several simple tasks that you know will generate "yes" or "I can" behaviors. Have the child engage successfully and reward the effort. Build a momentum of positive and "yes" behaviors, then present a less-preferred task and follow any effort with praise and reinforcement (Mace et al., 1988).

Vicky is four years old. She tantrums and slips out of the chair every time she has to do writing or coloring tasks. Behavioral momentum was used to get task compliance. Vicky's favorite activities revolve around Disney characters. Vicky was presented with a picture of her favorite Disney character on an incline board. She was asked questions she could answer: Who is this? Where are her ears? What's in her hair? What color should her eyes be? Let's color her eyes blue. Without thinking or questioning, she started coloring the eyes. Praise and reinforcement followed.

See appendix E for more information on environmental strategies.

Behavioral Intervention Techniques 8

Why Use Behavioral Intervention Strategies?

The goal of most intervention programs is to protect children from failure and help them build self-confidence and a sense of mastery over their environment. To give the child new skills and behaviors to replace ineffective ones, we must build his skills and give him more acceptable methods of getting his needs met. Once these new skills and behaviors are in place, we must give more attention to appropriate and on-task behaviors, rewarding the child for attempting to use them and convincing the child that these behaviors will work for him. Old, ineffective behaviors must be ignored. The new behaviors must receive more attention and rewards. This means that any fleeing or distracting behaviors must not result in task avoidance, tantrums must be ignored or made ineffective, and attempts to throw objects must be quietly redirected to a functional task.

Once we know the primary underlying cause of the behavior, it would be ideal to wait to see what happens as we work on the underlying problems, improving the child's coordination, strength, sensory-motor skills, sensory integration, and overall processing. However, the child can't wait until the underlying problem is addressed and therapy is effective. The child has developed ineffective coping strategies and challenging behaviors that interfere with therapy, learning, and living. Even if we are able to eliminate the behaviors and cure the underlying sensory, motor, communication, and learning problems, the child will not have the skills needed to be successful in his environment.

We must treat the underlying problem causing the challenging behavior, while giving the child coping strategies and behaviors that work *now*. This process involves a proactive approach. We must know which behaviors we want to develop and provide the child the tools, the environment, and the opportunities to practice these new behaviors and strategies. First, we must teach the child new coping strategies. Then, we must often use behavioral strategies to establish the new behaviors and extinguish the interfering behaviors that block the child's skill acquisition and active participation in therapy, school, home, and play. Intervening before the problem has occurred and using some basic behavioral strategies can help improve the quality of the child's interactions in all environments, resulting in quicker functional improvements.

Intervene Before the Challenging Behavior Occurs

Once the behavior is displayed, you must deal with it, which is usually exhausting and emotionally draining. On the other hand, if you are proactive, you can intervene before the behavior occurs and teach the child positive coping skills.

Proactive strategies focus on the child's positive, constructive, on-task behavior while ignoring or redirecting off-task behaviors.

Beginning, intermediate, and advanced professionals can be differentiated by their abilities to intercede before the behavior occurs. The *beginner* sees the behavior and tries to deal with it after it has occurred. The *intermediate* sees the warning signs for the behavior and as the child starts to escalate, intervenes. The *advanced* anticipates the behavior and either sets up the environment to prevent the behavior or intervenes in advance of the behavior. The result is that the child neither needs nor uses the behavior, but begins to explore coping strategies or alternative behaviors. In our drive to learn more, we are constantly striving to function at an advanced level, but may find ourselves unwittingly shifting between the beginner, intermediate, and advanced. It is not uncommon to change levels throughout the day. Each situation presents a new challenge. What's important is to not lose sight of the goal: helping the child function without ever needing the negative behavior.

The ultimate goal is to eliminate the need for the behavior. Our goal requires us to understand the child and why he behaves the way he does. Once we understand, we can develop a program that addresses the underlying cause for the behavior, and thereby eliminate the child's need to use it. We have learned that behaviors are often supported by more than one cause or factor. Even the best-designed programs frequently leave residual learned behaviors long after the underlying cause is removed. Behavioral strategies become important throughout the process to help the child function optimally (Murray-Slutsky and Paris 2000).

Table 8.1
Skill Levels in Dealing With Behavior

The Novice or Beginner
Allows the behavior to occur or attempts to stop or correct the behavior after it has occurred.
The Intermediate
Sees the warning signs of the behavior and as the behavior begins, intervenes.
The Advanced
Understands the behavior, anticipates it, and designs a program to prevent its need and occurrence.

What Behavior Do You Want to Occur?

The first step to using reinforcers is to know what behavior we want to reward. We have looked at what we don't want to occur, but it is equally important to identify what we *want* to occur. What is an acceptable response? The behavior the child displays is his *coping strategy*: how the child responds to situations and handles everyday activities and stress. The child often learns these strategies through trial and error. His coping strategies, though faulty, may be the only way he knows how to respond. Our job is to teach him different, more effective coping strategies. What behavior would we like to see?

Michel punched his uncle because he felt insulted. The strategy is to teach him to say, "I'm mad," and leave the room. In the other room he can use sensory strategies to calm himself down.

Kai pulls at his teacher's necklace and appears inappropriate. The strategy is to teach him to say, "It's a nice necklace," and get a fidget toy to keep his hands occupied.

Ana throws things or flees when she's had enough. The strategy is to teach her to say, "I'm done."

Mateo and Shaun are constantly fighting and arguing. The strategy is to teach them to play and work together.

Praise On-Task Behaviors and Ignore Negative Behaviors

Any behavior that is followed by a positive reinforcing consequence is more likely to happen again. Behaviors that are not rewarded or attended to will diminish in frequency (except sensory behaviors).

Don't take good behavior for granted. It is easy to focus on all the negative behaviors. Children believe what you tell them. If you tell a child he is sloppy because his room is not neat, he will believe it. Instead, if you tell a child: "You are not like this; you are a neater person than this," he will believe it. To change behavior, we must see every positive behavior the child does, as well as see the child in a positive light. Shine the spotlight on good behavior. Positive reinforcement is the most powerful tool we have to change behavior, to improve the child's self esteem, and to give a motivational boost.

Give specific praise and use the child's name. By hearing his name, the child will start to associate it with positive activities. Specific praise leaves no room for speculation about what it was that you liked. For example, Chris finishes his writing paper and throws his papers on the floor. At the same time you say, "Good boy." What was good? Chris completing his writing paper or throwing the paper on the floor? If you had said, "Chris, I like how you finished your paper so neatly," he would have clearly known what he did correctly and you would not have inadvertently reinforced negative behavior.

When Michael tells his uncle, "I'm mad," and leaves the room, tell him, "Michael, you should be so proud of yourself. That was the perfect way to handle the situation."

When Kai admires the teacher's necklace and keeps his hands to himself, tell him, "Kai, thank you. That is such a nice thing for you to say."

When Ana says, "All done," rather than throwing her activity or fleeing, tell her, "Ana, that was great talking."

When you see Mateo help Shaun, say, "Mateo, you are helping Shaun. That is such a nice thing for you to do."

Empower children with your praise. Children believe what you tell them. If you tell them they are sloppy or lazy, they will believe you. Your words have the power to build up a child's self-esteem and confidence. Stop looking for negative behaviors. Become a detective and uncover the good behaviors. If you catch them doing something right, tell them. For example: "You are so neat. Look at how you put your pencil in the correct place. That is great."

Table 8.2
Treatment Strategies to Facilitate Positive Outcomes in Learning

Identify the target behavior	Identify the behavior you want to occur, not the challenging behavior you want to stop.
Attend to "on-task" behavior	Give more attention to on-task behaviors than to negative behaviors.
	Provide reinforcement every time the new behavior is displayed.
Avoid punishment and reprimands	Avoid negative attention, verbal reprimands, or punishments because they will reward the exact behavior you are trying to stop.

(continued)

Table 8.2 Treatment Strategies to Facilitate Positive Outcomes in Learning (*Continued*)

Reinforcers	Identify the targeted behavior and the appropriate reinforcer.
	Use rewards and forms of reinforcement that are motivating to the child.
	Reinforce only the targeted behavior. Reinforce the targeted behavior immediately, once it is displayed.
	Reinforce the targeted behavior consistently, every time it is displayed.
	Grade reinforcers from primary to secondary and from consistent to intermittent.
	Remember that in order to function independently, a child must be internally motivated and respond to secondary reinforcers, such as praise, on an intermittent basis. Progress to use of intermittent secondary reinforcers to promote independence.
Delay gratification or reinforcement	Teach the child to tolerate delayed gratification or reinforcement while continuing to work.
	Wait until just before the child reaches his maximum level; present a concrete end to the task, slightly beyond his or her tolerance, then provide reinforcement.
Prompt or facilitate the desired behavior	**Never use prompts until you know the child's baseline functioning without prompts or assistance.**
	Physical prompts or facilitation — Physically assist or guide the child through the activity.
	Visual prompts — Provide visual cues, drawings, symbols, or written rules or instructions that assist the child to remember or sequence the task.
	Demonstration — Demonstrate the desired response while the child imitates it. This requires that the child have a good sensory-motor concept of his body.
	Modeling — Have one child model the desired response for another child.
	Auditory or verbal prompts — Assist the child with verbal directions. Prompts may also be given by varying volume and inflections.
	Combine prompts to gradually decrease the assistance provided.
Shape the response	Use this technique to teach a behavior or skill that is not in the child's repertoire.
	Forward Chaining — Task is broken into component parts. Child is taught to independently perform the steps, from the first to the last, in a forward progression.
	Backwards Chaining — Task is broken into the component parts. Child is taught to independently perform the steps, from the last to the first (works backwards).
Use time-outs	***Request a Time-Out*** — Teach the child with sensory overload, anxiety, or regulatory disorders to take time-out to reorganize.
	Keep atmosphere positive and compassionate.
	Give a Nonpunitive Time-Out — Remove the child from the environment (reinforcer) and do one of the following:
	■ Do not talk to, make eye contact with, or attend to the child.
	■ Give an exercise time-out. Use heavy work to calm and reorganize.
	■ Coach the child through calming strategies.
	Adult Time-Out — Use this technique to interrupt attention-seeking challenging behaviors in order to reward appropriate behavior. Stop and shut down all activity, averting gaze for fifteen to twenty seconds, then reward next appropriate behavior.

Reinforcers

Changing how a child behaves relies on reinforcers. Almost everything we do has a consequence. When we engage in an activity that has a positive consequence (reinforcement), we are more likely to repeat the activity. Most of us work for a paycheck or the satisfaction we receive from what we do. If the reinforcer was altered and we stopped receiving a paycheck or stopped receiving satisfaction from our work, would we continue? What is the reinforcing factor that you work for?

What motivates someone is uniquely individual. We must identify a reward that the child finds motivating and pleasing. If the child does not value the reward, the behavior will not be established. For some children, primary reinforcers, those with inherent rewards (such as a certain food or a sensory experience) will need to be used. For others, secondary reinforcers such as praise or adult attention will be sufficient. To identify what is motivating to a child:

- ask people who know the child well for his preferred activities,

- observe what the child chooses during free time,

- ask the child his preferred reward,

- present several options and ask the child to choose, or

- present various reinforcers and see how the child responds.

By observing the child's response (positive or negative) and behavior (increased or decreased compliance), you can develop a list of reinforcers that work.

Children who derive their rewards from *negative attention* require a thorough evaluation of what component of that negative attention reinforces the behavior. Is it the strength of handling, as when an adult grabs the child by the arm, or is it a chase that ensues as the adult races after the child? Is it the one-to-one attention, the darting glance, or the shocked reaction the child gets from an adult, or is it the reactions of the other children around? Make a list of what you think is motivating the child.

The reinforcers we choose must have the same intensity, duration, and frequency as the reinforcer that is supporting the undesirable behavior. This is often hard to do. Giving firm, forceful negative attention is easy, and it usually draws attention from others, which further reinforces the behavior. We must instead give equally firm, forceful attention in praise of the desired behavior. Analyze the components of the negative behavior that the child finds rewarding and incorporate similar characteristics into the praise, being sure to match the intensity level the child craves. The sensory input of firm handling, the shock reaction, or your fast movements toward the child can be used positively.

It is important to remember that you are a part of the child's environment and that your reaction or attention to his behavior may serve either as a primary cause or a secondary reinforcer to sustain the behavior you want to eliminate.

You must deal with the child calmly; not with anger. As the child's behavior escalates, the quieter, slower, and calmer your responses need to be. *Do not allow yourself to escalate as the child's behavior erupts.*

When teaching a new skill or establishing a new behavior (to replace the undesirable behavior), reinforcement should occur after every desired response. As the child's performance improves, reinforcement should be reduced to every second or third response (intermittently). Start with primary reinforcers, if needed at first, and then move to secondary reinforcers as the child learns the value of praise and positive attention. To teach the value of a secondary reinforcer, such as praise, use it simultaneously with the primary reinforcer. Gradually decrease the primary reinforcer, using only praise or other secondary reinforcers. Start by giving praise to every positive occurrence and gradually decrease it to every third or fourth occurrence (intermittently).

Use of Primary Reinforcers

Developing a new behavior is extremely labor intensive and time consuming. Reinforcers must be given every time the desired behavior occurs. Rewards for that behavior must be strong enough to promote repeated use of the new behavior. Primary reinforcers are those that are inherently rewarding and result in behavioral changes. Preferred food items are common and effective, if used correctly. The food item must be broken into small pieces to not satiate the appetite and lessen the food's effectiveness.

Research has shown that obsessive behaviors, objects, and toys are actually primary reinforcers, and that engaging in these behaviors is inherently reinforcing. Brief use, three to five seconds, of the object of obsession has been effective in increasing learning, and if paired with the desired behavior, will increase its frequency.

Many children also find sensory-based activities such as swinging or jumping are strong primary reinforcers and can be even stronger reinforcers than food or drink. Depending on the child's preference, roughhousing, jumping on a trampoline, resistive exercise equipment (clothespins or grippers), bubble gum, or music may be helpful. Matching the sensory-based activity to the child's specific sensory needs makes the activity not only reinforcing but therapeutic. For a child who craves proprioceptive input (into the joints) or vestibular input (movement), jumping on a trampoline, being thrown in the air, and swinging are primary reinforcers. A child with decreased sensory feedback into his hands may like resistive clothespins. Children who find sounds reinforcing enjoy having sounds paired with movement (for example, vocalizations paired with pencil strokes). Singing and rhythmic activities are primary reinforcers for many children. Through carefully analyzing what the child chooses during his free time, the type of sensory-based activities he finds enjoyable, and looking at his overall sensory needs, we can develop a list of sensory-based activities that are reinforcing.

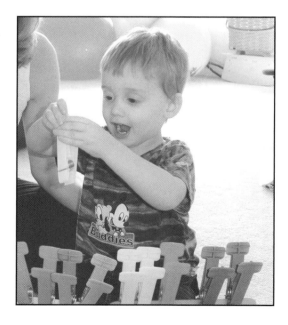

For underresponsive children, resistive clothespins can be primary reinforcers because of the sensory feedback they provide.

Identifying the primary reinforcer for a child is an individualized process that involves more than just making a list of the child's favorite foods and activities. It involves finding reinforcers that are effective in increasing the desired behavior. A common mistake parents and professionals make is to assume that a child's favorite activity or food is an effective reinforcer. A reinforcer is only effective if it increases the desired behavior. Therefore, a child may love hugs, jumping on a trampoline, or a particular candy or toy, but if it is not effective in increasing the desired behavior, it is not a reinforcer.

Preferred reinforcers are primary reinforcers with the strongest reward potential, and therefore, the greatest impact on behavioral change. Reinforcers come in all strengths, and some have more reinforcing potential than others. To identify preferred reinforcers, Maurice, Green, and Luce (1996) recommend selecting a few potentially reinforcing objects and presenting them to the child one by one. Objects that are preferred are:

1. Those that the child plays with for more than fifteen seconds without encouragement (or eats readily if you are using food).

2. Those that the child resists having taken away.

3. Those that the child will try to get back when they are placed about a foot away.

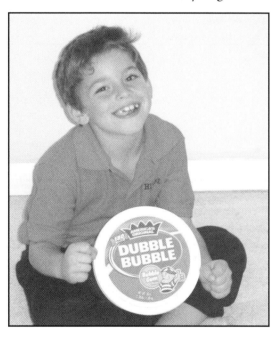

Bubble gum is a strong reinforcer for an underresponsive child, in that it provides proprioceptive input.

Use of Secondary Reinforcers

Secondary reinforcers are those that the child has learned to appreciate. Praise, attention, a favorite DVD or video, touch or tickling, stickers, smiley faces, tokens, and money are but a few examples. For the young child, a favorite toy might be a secondary reinforcer. The toy is given to the child for a few seconds, taken back while the child works, and given once again to the child when he completes a set or the entire task. This process is then repeated with the next activity or task.

It is important that children be moved from primary to secondary reinforcers. The most convenient, easily available form of secondary reinforcement is praise. It can be given at any time without preparation. To teach the value of a secondary reinforcer such as praise, use it simultaneously with the primary reinforcer. For example, if your primary reinforcer is a small piece of candy, every time the child gives the correct answer he receives the candy, plus the secondary reinforcer, "Great answer!" As the child progresses, continue to give the secondary reinforcer, "Great answer!" every time he responds correctly, while giving the candy with the praise on every third or fourth correct response. Gradually decrease the primary reinforcer (candy), leaving only verbal praise or other secondary reinforcers. Eventually decrease the use of the secondary reinforcer (praise) by giving praise intermittently, to every third or fourth occurrence of positive behavior.

Grading the Reinforcers

Our goal is to help children succeed, to build their self-confidence, and to give them a sense of mastery over their environment. This requires tapping into their internal motivation and drive, and consistent use of external rewards may interfere with achieving this goal.

Table 8.3
Grading Reinforcers

Apply reinforcers to correct responses or desired behaviors. Grade the reinforcers from the most concentrated and intense motivators to the least.

Primary reinforcer, consistently administered, with secondary reinforcer consistently administered

Secondary reinforcer, administered consistently with primary reinforcer, administered every third or fourth response

Secondary reinforcer administered consistently

Secondary reinforcer administered every third or fourth correct response (intermittent)

Developing new behaviors requires consistent administration of primary reinforcers. You will need to use the child's preferred reinforcers, giving the child extra motivation for learning and engaging in new behaviors. To establish the new behavior, you must reinforce the behavior every time it occurs, in every environment (consistently), or it will not be established. This new behavior must draw more attention and be more intensely rewarded and at a greater frequency than the behavior you are trying to extinguish.

Maintaining a new behavior once it is established is much easier and less demanding than developing new behaviors. Intermittent reinforcement, the strongest form of reinforcement, of a secondary reinforcer (praise) is effective in maintaining the behavior and in activating the child's internal motivation and drive.

Rewards and reinforcers are also a method of helping children through difficult or new tasks. As the workload intensifies or when introducing a new skill, you may have to revert to using a primary reinforcer initially, while using a secondary reinforcer for familiar tasks. It is not a regression to move from secondary to primary reinforcers when activities are harder, new to the child, or the environment changes or is more challenging. Reinforcers frequently need to be altered based on the activity the child engages in or the environment in which the child must function.

Primary reinforcers may be needed to reward a child for performing tasks that are necessary but not intrinsically rewarding, like dressing, writing, or speaking. For example, a child not driven to speak will not be intrinsically motivated to repeat words or make verbal utterances. Primary reinforcers of desirable sensory experiences or food may be linked to repeating sounds or words. Once the child produces the desired response, it can be linked to both the primary reinforcer and secondary reinforcer (praise).

Delayed Gratification

Behaviors are often the expression of a need for immediate gratification. Therefore, teaching delayed gratification, or a delay in reinforcement, can often be effective in warding off undesirable behavior and expanding the child's tolerance for work. This technique is often used with a child who displays attention-seeking or avoidance behaviors. Examples of children who need to learn delayed gratification include:

- Children who display "full-ownership" behaviors with their parents or teacher, refusing to allow them to talk with other adults.

- Children who quickly reach their frustration tolerance with a task, then revert to avoidance behaviors.

- Children who demonstrate attention-seeking ploys.

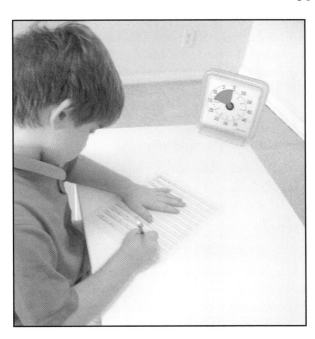

The Time Timer™ presents a visual depiction of time and can clearly define the amount of time the child must work before the next transition.

Delayed gratification of reinforcements involves first identifying the warning signs of escalating behavior. Learn to recognize the child's tolerance and frustration level, and then intercede immediately before the behavior erupts. Your intervention always includes praise or primary reinforcers for work well done, followed by a command to either extend the work or the waiting time.

For example:

- If the child displays "full ownership" and will not allow you to interact with others, have the child play quietly with a toy while you interact with an adult. At the child's maximum tolerance level or warning signs of unrest, go over and praise the child (or use a primary reinforcer) and have the child play quietly for another specified period of time, extending the original waiting time.

- For the child who needs to expand his work tolerance or displays avoidance behaviors, have the child complete his work to his maximum capacity, and/or to the point at which he displays the warning signs of escalating behaviors, then intervene. Praise the child for his good work, then delay the gratification (reinforcement) by telling him he only has three more to do, then he gets a reward (or break). Remove all items from in front of the child, except the three remaining items.

In each case, gradually increase the amount of time the child must wait or the amount of items the child must complete before the child gets a break or gets to end the task. Reward on-task behavior and give positive reinforcement when the child completes the task and you release him.

Teaching tolerance for delayed gratification is also an effective method of teaching a child self-awareness and socially acceptable ways to communicate these feelings. First set up the situation so that the behavior will occur. Intervene at the warning signs, before the behavior is displayed. Your intervention involves exploring with the child how he is feeling and what he needs. Help the child label his feelings correctly and to request the appropriate action. Remember to be specific when facilitating the communication request and rewarding the appropriate behavioral response. When the child effectively communicates what he feels and needs, it is critical that you reward the child by giving the requested activity. After he receives it, you may then re-engage him in the original activity and continue the process. Examples might include:

- The child is tired and needs a break.

- The child is hot and needs a drink/break.

- The child is bored and wants to do something else.

Remember that when teaching a new skill or behavior, every correct response must be reinforced until the behavior is established.

Use Time-Outs Constructively

Time-outs are often used in a negative way as a form of punishment; the child is placed in time-out after he has done something wrong or has displayed bad behavior. When time-out is used for the purpose of punishment, it is usually an attempt to *suppress* negative behaviors. Several problems occur when using aversive activities for the purpose of punishment: First, they have been proven to be ineffective in creating behavioral changes in all environments, and second, it has been proven that it is easier to teach new skills and behaviors rather than attempt to suppress or punish unwanted behaviors. In addition, punishment sometimes elicits additional disruptive behavior, such as emotional outbursts or escape or avoidance behavior (Favell and Greene 1981; Luce and Christian 1981). Time-outs for the purpose of punishment also lower the child's self-esteem and often reinforce avoidance behaviors by allowing the child to avoid or escape a task, person, or activity. *Time-outs used as a punishment should be discouraged.*

There are three types of therapeutic time-outs.

Giving a nonpunitive time-out. The nonpunitive time-out removes the child from the environment that contains the reinforcers and allows the child time to regain control over his emotions and behaviors. The child is moved only a short distance from the activity, just far enough to interrupt the reinforcer. During the time-out, one of the following things can occur:

- No one talks to the child, makes eye contact with the child, or attends to any ploys to get attention.

- Give an exercise time-out. The child is given heavy work such as push-ups, pull-ups, handstands, or wheelbarrow exercises that provide proprioception and are organizing. This bottom-up approach helps the child organize from the inside-out by utilizing calming sensory strategies.

- Coach the child through the calming process. Teach the child techniques that are calming and organizing, such as deep breathing, counting slowly, closing his eyes, and consciously trying to reorganize. With this top-down approach, the child learns cognitive strategies to regain control and to display appropriate behaviors.

Remember that the time-out must be used constructively and with positive connotations. It is a method of getting the child out of a situation or environment, giving the child time to reorganize and the adult the opportunity to reward the appropriate behavior. It is not meant as a form of punishment. Your vocal quality and volume must remain calm.

Requesting to take a time-out is an effective coping strategy when a child needs to self-regulate. Adults utilize this coping method to get away from a task for a moment, to decrease stress in their everyday life, and to gather their thoughts before proceeding. A child who is experiencing anxiety or sensory overload from the environment must have time to take a break and reorganize himself. When a child is escalating, becoming overwhelmed or out of control, a time-out can give him the edge he needs to regroup and organize. Increasing the child's self-awareness, teaching him to recognize signs of escalating stress, anxiety, and overarousal, is the first step in teaching self-regulation.

Visual aids may be used within a behavioral program to teach self-awareness. Use of the stoplight has been helpful. Green indicates, "You are doing well;" yellow means, "Your behavior is escalating;" and red may indicate, "Take a time-out." The goal of this approach is to teach the child to recognize the signs of escalating behaviors (yellow) and learn to intervene before needing a time-out (red).

Programs such as *How Does Your Engine Run*, the Alert Program, by Shellenberger and Williams, are designed to improve awareness of self-regulation and to guide children to recognize hypersensitivities affecting them. The Alert Program and their book, *Take Five*, help children learn strategies to change their levels of alertness and arousal.

One of the goals of having a child request a time-out is to empower the child to change his arousal level and behavior. Part of empowering the child involves encouraging him to initiate requests for self-regulation time-outs, as well as allowing him to be involved in choosing where the time-out will be taken.

An *adult time-out* is used to interrupt attention-seeking problem behaviors. The adult stops what he or she is doing, freezing in place, and *averting the eye gaze* from the child for fifteen to twenty seconds. This technique is effective when working closely with a child who uses attention-getting behaviors that are difficult to ignore. By shutting down and averting your gaze, you wait for an interruption in the child's behavior to reinforce quiet behavior. It is important to reward the on-task behavior at the next opportunity. Since quiet, on-task behavior is what you are looking for, if you receive it within the fifteen to twenty seconds of time-out, discontinue the time-out and reward the behavior.

Time-outs lasting longer than twenty seconds or direct eye contact during the time-out will reinforce the challenging behavior you are trying to interrupt.

If a child displays a behavior in an attempt to avoid work and is given a time-out that allows him to get out of the work, the time-out will reinforce the avoidance behavior. Monitor time-outs carefully to assure that they are not reinforcing task avoidance.

Use Positive Behavioral Momentum

Positive behavioral momentum is a strategy that encourages "yes" answers and minimizes negative responses. Positive behavioral momentum builds the child's self-esteem and gives the child self-confidence. Because the targeted task is buried within a series of positive rewarding activities, the child complies without ever realizing it is a less desirable task. It is a perfect way to avoid power struggles or "no" answers. Start with several simple tasks that you know will generate "yes" or "I can" behaviors. Have the child successfully engage, and reward the effort. After building a momentum of positive and "yes" behaviors, present a less preferred task. Follow any effort on the less desirable task with praise and reinforcement (Mace et al. 1988; Cipani 1998).

Getting Mireya dressed and ready to go to school in the morning is a strenuous feat resulting in her screaming and running through the house to avoid being caught. The morning usually starts with Mireya having breakfast, watching TV, and then getting ready for school (the fight). The sequence was changed to assure positive behavioral momentum and compliance. In her room, after awaking, she was asked "Do you want to have breakfast?" "Are you hungry"? "Do you want to watch TV?" Each question received a "yes" answer. Enthusiastically, the next statement was "Let's get your shirt on, pants, then socks."

Jacobs' first answer to everything is "no." The targeted behavior is to put his lunch box away. He is told, "Give me five," "Give me a hug," "Show me your hands," "Put your lunch box away."

Darrel had a tantrum in the hallway. Even though it has subsided he refuses to go into class. Paying attention to his behavior and addressing it head-on results in more defiance. Positive behavioral intervention worked. He was asked, "How old are you?" followed by: "Count to ten," "Slap me five," "Give me a hug," "What's your favorite animal?" "Stand up," "Walk into class."

Use of Prompts to Facilitate Desired Behavior

Some children need extra help to perform the desired skill or behavior so that you can reinforce it. Prompting or facilitating a child's response is an effective technique to assist the child in understanding and performing in a desired manner. A variety of prompts may be used depending on the skill and understanding of the child. These include physical, visual, or verbal prompts; modeling; demonstration; gesturing; or shaping. Consistency in all environments is critical to the success of prompting. All people working with the child must follow the same methods and prompts. If cues or prompts and teaching methods are not consistent, the child may not learn the desired behavior.

Physical Prompts

Physical prompting, in which the adult physically assists and guides the child, may vary from hand-over-hand (full physical assistance) to intermittently guiding a child in a movement, to a light touch at the shoulder to initiate a response (partial assistance). Full hand-over-hand assistance is effective in teaching children tasks that are totally unfamiliar to them. With assistance, children can experience the end result and will begin to understand the process of getting there: Hand-over-hand assistance connects the activity with the end result and assists with motor planning, ideation, and skill development. Intermittently guiding a child assumes he understands some of the steps needed to complete the activity. When the child falters, physical assistance is provided to assure continued success and involvement in the activity.

Children who have difficulty understanding or who have auditory processing difficulties are easily overwhelmed and frustrated by auditory stimulation and verbal instructions. These children often respond well to, and appreciate, physical prompting and gestures. Physical prompts help the child know what the words mean. If the child understands but chooses not to respond, the physical guidance teaches that you expect him to comply. Physical prompts can be as simple as asking the child to sit down while gently putting pressure on the child's shoulder in the direction of sitting or as complex as physically prompting a child through the cafeteria line.

Physical prompts are effective in modifying self-stimulation behaviors without directing attention to or negatively reinforcing the behavior. Self-stimulatory behaviors that are repetitive, that block the child's engagement and function, or that are socially inappropriate should be redirected. Extinguish self-stimulation behaviors (such as obsessions with small objects and strings, hand flapping, fingering objects, or hand wringing) by not reacting, removing the object, providing some other activity, or redirecting the hands into productive positions and responses. Reward appropriate behavior immediately. Remember, self-stimulation behaviors often have a sensory component that reinforces the behavior. A sensory program is needed in addition to physical prompts. (Refer to sensory-obtaining behaviors—nonproductive in chapter 5.)

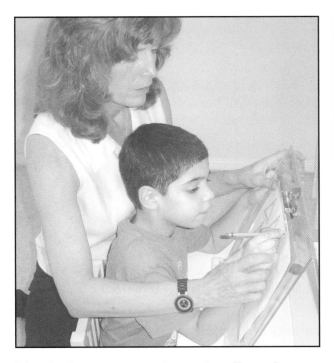

Physical prompts at the wrist allow the child to independently complete the parts of the task he knows. When the child falters, physical assistance is provided to assure continued success.

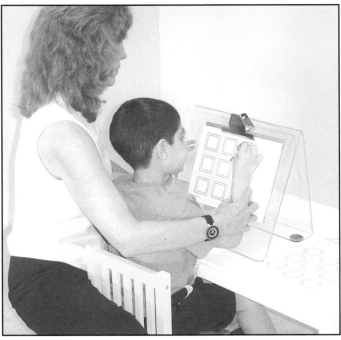

Moving the physical prompt to the forearm fades the prompt and requires the child to work more independently.

Fading Prompts

Physical prompts need to be gradually faded until the child can independently complete the desired activity. Fading is accomplished through gradually decreasing the amount of physical assistance provided. Maurice, Green, and Luce (1996) describe techniques to fade physical assistance:

- Gradually decrease the amount of physical effort you exert to help the child respond, lightening your handhold on the child and gradually applying less and less pressure.

- Gradually move the physical prompt away from the hand, progressing to the wrist, forearm, elbow, and so on, until it is no longer needed.

- *Most-to-least prompting.* Begin with a full physical prompt, then fade to a gesture or model and end with verbal instructions. This is an excellent technique for teaching brand-new skills.

- *Least-to-most prompting.* Give the child the opportunity to respond independently, then after a brief delay, gradually provide assistance (verbal prompt—model—physical prompt) until the child responds appropriately.

- *Time delay.* Fade the prompt gradually by increasing the intervals of time between the instruction and the delivery of the physical or verbal prompt.

Visual Prompts

Visual prompts provide less assistance than physical prompts. Visual prompts may include:

- Visually cuing the child to the correct response, such as pointing to the correct response or in the general area of the correct response.

- Cuing the child to visually scan the answers by scanning your finger from left to right across the page (gesturing).

- Visually placing the correct answer closer to the child to increase the likelihood he may pick it (positional cue). For example, ask the child to point to the picture of the horse; place the horse closer to the child than the other pictures.

- Physically gesturing the meaning of a word (such as stand up or sit down).

- Visually glancing in the direction of the child to keep him on task.

- Using pictures depicting activities and schedules.

Written instructions, rules posted on a wall, schedules written on the board, and pictures that depict the next activity are all examples of visual prompts that help remind the child of what he needs to do. The picture may depict skills the child needs to practice. Visuals are an effective way of transforming abstract concepts into more concrete images. They can be effective as a method of teaching self-monitoring and self-awareness.

Steven's occupational therapist is frustrated by his lack of compliance. Sessions have become battlegrounds in which Steven refuses to comply with any request, even if it is clearly within his capability. In the past, Steven used task refusal as a method of coping with decreased processing skills. He did not understand what was being asked of him, so he would say "No, I don't want to do this; I want to do that." By controlling both the request and the activity, he could assure that he both understood the request and that he could complete the activity. He learned to link negative responses with "whining" behaviors, reverting to the latter when "no" did not work.

Steven's behavior is now a learned response that occurs automatically and spontaneously following any request or demand. It is interfering with his learning to improve his processing skills and his functional skills. The negative tension is also counterproductive and interferes with his internal motivation and drive. The therapist is working on decreasing Steven's negative and whining behaviors while improving his self-awareness and self-monitoring. A scoreboard-type sign is posted above Steven's workstation. He is asked to begin a task. He impulsively responds "no." Without attending to his negative behavior a mark is placed in the "no" column. The task is reintroduced. Steven retorts, "No, I don't want to," and the therapist places another mark under the "no" column without emotion or a sense of punishment. By the fourth time Steven responds with whining. The therapist asks, "Did I hear whining?" and describes whining behavior. The therapist moves a hand toward the "whining" column as if to mark it. Steven yells out, "No, don't mark it. It's not whining. I said, 'I want to do it.' " The therapist repeats: "You want to do it. That's wonderful!" and moves away from the sign, rewarding the appropriate behavior. By the end of the session, the therapist only has to move in the direction of marking the sign to serve as a visual reminder of the desired behavior. Steven monitors what he is saying, stopping mid-sentence to self-correct, saying, "I'd love to do it."

Responding with "no" or whining was an automatic learned response that helped Steven cope when he could not process the instructions. Now he has the skills to process the instructions, but he still responds automatically to avert the task. By extinguishing the learned response, Steven was forced to process the verbal instructions. He realized that he understood the request and that he had the skills needed to do the activity. What appeared to be lack of task compliance was actually learned behaviors.

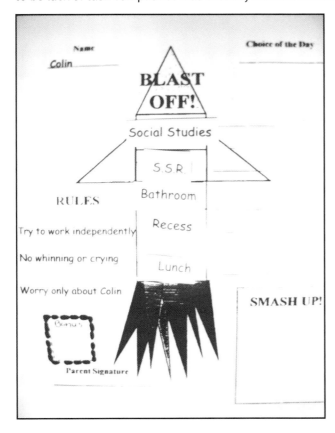

Token charts can positively reward a child for desired behaviors.

In the classroom, teachers often list or post pictures of desirable behaviors. The children have matching lists or pictures on their desks, and the teacher gives smiley faces when any of the children display the desired behavior. Rewarded behaviors include sitting quietly in place, raising their hands, keeping hands to themselves, and not talking. Stop signs may be used at hallways where children need to stop and line up, providing visual cues for behaviors (Murray-Slutsky and Paris 2000).

Demonstration and Modeling

Modeling consists of actually demonstrating the correct response for children and asking them to follow the model. A child can only benefit from modeling if he can imitate. Imitating the body movements of others requires good sensorimotor awareness of their bodies and how they move and relate to their environment.

Modeling a desired response can also be accomplished by using the child's peers. A child with stronger fine motor skills may be paired with a child who needs to acquire these skills, using the more accomplished child as a model. Rewarding the desired behavior in both children is critical. Positively reinforce the child who is modeling the correct response, drawing attention to the specific behavior you want modeled ("Henry, I love how you are holding the pencil!"). If the second child requires physical prompts, provide them until he displays the desired behavior, then give specific praise immediately ("Carlos, your two fingers on the pencil are perfect!"). When using peers for modeling, it is important to keep the atmosphere positive and empowering, especially for the child with the lower skills. The goal is not to have one child teach the other, but to have them learn from each other as equals. Rewarding each child for his individual contributions and strengths sets the environment for positive interactions.

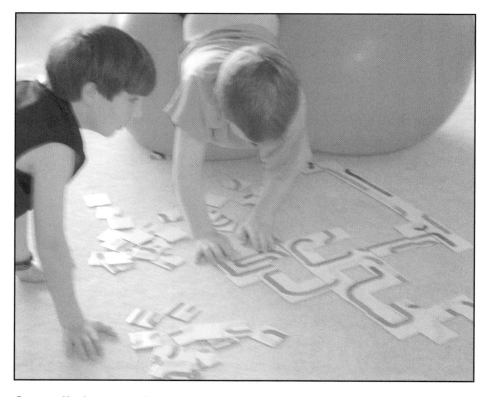

Controlled competition can be a strong reinforcer.

Controlled Competition

Building in controlled competition can be a strong reinforcer to modeling. Many children thrive with a little bit of competition, demonstrating increased enthusiasm and motivation. Competition can be set up in nonthreatening ways—without having a loser—while motivating and modeling the desired behaviors and responses. Positive competition, if the child believes he can do the task, will drive the child to succeed. Controlled competition may include:

- Team two children up on one team.
    - Have them work together to get correct answers.
    - Have each child take turns doing a similar task. Each time, ask who wants to go first. As the child with the weaker skills learns how to respond (models the behavior), he will start to request to go first.

- Have two children work at the same time on two different activities. Have the children compete to finish their own task correctly, making sure they cannot compare their results. Switch tasks.

- Have a child compete against his own score. Get a baseline of the child's performance on a task, and then see if he can beat it. Record the child's scores and progress. Repeat the process.

- Have the child compete against children not present at the time. Record the names of other children, their scores, and their age or grade. Compare the child's score with that of children he does not know.

- Have the child compete against the adult.

Verbal Prompts and Verbal Feedback

Verbal instructions can easily overwhelm a child. Weak auditory processing, auditory figure ground, auditory defensiveness, or receptive language skills can make verbal instructions confusing and overwhelming. Verbal instructions are abstract, and once given, they are lost in time and space. Remember to keep the number of verbal instructions to a minimum. Combine verbal instructions with visual cues, gestures, and physical prompts to aid the child in understanding the instructions. Offer physical or visual prompts initially, and gradually move to more abstract, intermittent prompts, such as verbal cues alone.

Voice volume and inflection are important when using verbal prompts. By changing your voice volume or inflection, you can emphasize parts of the conversation the child is missing or needs to focus on. "Give me your *hand*," "Give *me* your hand," "Place *your backpack* in the cubby," "Place your backpack *in the cubby*," are examples of how changes in inflection can be used as cues or prompts. Your command or request must emphasize the words you want the child to focus on.

Children who have difficulty understanding verbal instructions often comprehend only the noun or the noun and the verb, not all the words in between. "Give me the ball," often translates initially into "Ball." The child does not initially understand what you want him to do with the ball. Gestures, physical prompts, visual cues, and modeling may be necessary to teach the child what to do with the ball. Placing more inflection on the verb, "*Give* me the ball," will then translate into, "Give ball." If you then change the command to, "Give me the big ball," the child may not understand which ball and hand you the nearest ball. You can use inflection to denote which ball to give by saying, "Give me the *big* ball."

It is sometimes necessary to provide verbal consequences following a behavior to make it less likely to occur. For example, some children may be corrected, told "no," or redirected after an incorrect response. Scientific literature would define these actions as punishments. Consequences do not need to be aversive, appear to be negative, or provoke discomfort. In some cases, children may benefit when they are corrected or told "no" when they give the wrong response. The behavioral technique of ignoring the wrong answer, waiting for the correct answer to occur, and then delivering the reinforcer works for some children. Others respond very well to a more direct approach of correcting their behavior.

When a child tunes out auditory information, the brain is saying that information is not important to attend to. This often signals a problem with sensory registration, or difficulty registering or processing auditory information. Changes in voice volume and inflection help children who tune out or do not attend to auditory information. Linking exaggerated verbal and gestural prompts can further enhance the child's ability to register the auditory input.

Shaping

Shaping is a technique used to teach a behavior or skill that the child has not yet learned. It is particularly helpful in teaching a task in which steps are performed in a particular sequence, such as most dressing and self-help skills. It involves breaking the task into its various steps or components and teaching one component at a time, building upon previous knowledge. Sometimes it is helpful to write down the steps and post them where the activity takes place, such as hand-washing techniques or bathroom procedures above the sink. This provides a verbal prompt and encourages consistent implementation.

If you choose to start from step one and build, you would be using a technique termed forward chaining. Have the child independently master the first step in the chain while you prompt or assist later steps. For example, you may have the child put on his shirt by pulling it over his head independently, and then use physical prompts to get his arms into the sleeves and pull the shirt down. Later you would have the child independently pull the shirt over his head and push one arm through a sleeve, prompt the second arm into the sleeve, and pull the shirt down. You continue teaching or chaining the steps until the child can perform the process independently.

Conversely, *backward chaining* uses the chaining principle but teaches the child the last step to completion as a first step. In teaching the child to put on his shirt, the adult would pull the shirt over the child's head, assist his arms through the sleeves, and teach the child to pull the shirt down as a last step, independently. Then the adult would pull the shirt over the child's head, assist one arm through the sleeve, and have the child place the second arm through the sleeve and pull the shirt down. The teaching process continues until all steps are mastered and the child can put on his shirt independently. The advantage to this type of instruction is that the child's reward is in the successful task completion. It is especially useful with the child who is afraid of failure and believes that he cannot accomplish the task. The child gets immediate success for his efforts.

Approximating the desired response is a shaping technique that involves rewarding any response that approximates the desired behavior. You reward any movement in the correct direction, gradually asking for closer and closer approximations to the desired response. Eventually, you reward only the desired response. For example, Gabriel is currently able to gesture his wants and needs. We would like him to be verbally able to request activities. When he gestures we teach him the words he needs. Initially we reward *any* verbalization connected to a physical gesture requesting an activity, whether it matches our verbalizations or not. Gradually we require closer and closer approximations to the modeled word, progressing until Gabriel independently requests activities verbally. Shaping and reinforcement strategies are used together to achieve the desired goal. Shaping requires a great deal of patience, often taking weeks to months to achieve the desired response.

Summary of Behavioral Strategies

Give the child coping strategies and behaviors that work *now*. A child has a need to obtain or avoid something in the here and now. We cannot ask the child to wait while we build skills, improve sensory issues, and increase self-esteem. Being proactive, intervening before the behavior occurs, while using some basic behavioral strategies can result in quicker improvements.

Identify the behaviors you want to stop and ignore them.

Intervene before the behavior occurs.

- Create an environment in which the child does not need the behavior.

- Intervene at the warning signs.

- Proactive strategies focus on the child's positive, constructive, on-task behaviors while ignoring or redirecting negative, nonproductive, off-task behaviors.

Identify the behavior you want to occur.

- Attend to and reward or praise on-task behavior. Use reinforcement every time the new behavior is displayed.

- Avoid punishment or verbal reprimands. Do not ask the child why he did something. Remember, negative attention rewards the behavior.

- Reinforce the targeted behavior immediately.

  - Only use reinforcers that the child finds motivating or pleasurable. If the child does not value the reinforcer, or if the reinforcer does not result in behavioral change (no matter what you think of it) eliminate its use.

  - Move from a primary reinforcer to a secondary reinforcer as quickly as the child will respond to the secondary reinforcer.

  - Make intermittent use of a secondary reinforcer such as praise your goal. Intermittent reinforcement sustains behaviors.

- Teach the child to tolerate delays in gratification and reinforcement.

- Increase the child's level of performance.

  - Determine the child's previous performance level.

  - Establish a target by increasing performance expectations by approximately one or two.

  - Convey the new target to the child: "Today we will do ten."

  - Reward task completion with a reinforcer.

- Use prompts to extend a child's baseline performance.

  - Physical prompts or facilitation provide physical assistance to guide the child through an activity.

  - Visual prompts consist of visual cues, drawings, symbols, written lists, or instructions to assist the child in sequencing a task.

  - Modeling or demonstration provides cues for the child to imitate. This requires the child to know how to imitate and that the child have sufficient body scheme and awareness to imitate what is demonstrated.

  - Auditory or verbal prompts are verbal directions.

  - Prompts can be combined at first to tap multiple sensory systems and should be faded so as not to make the child prompt-dependent.

- Shaping the response teaches a child a behavior or response not already in his repertoire.

  - Forward chaining is a method of teaching that breaks the task into component parts. The child is taught one step at a time, from first to last.

  - Backward chaining teaches the child to perform the steps independently from the last to the first. Example: In shoe tying, the adult may do all the tying, but ask the child to pull the laces tight. Once the child has mastered the last step, he is asked to assist with the step that comes before pulling the laces tight, and so on.

- Use time-outs to your advantage.

  - A nonpunitive time-out removes the child from the environment that contains the reinforcement. Do not use this time-out as a type of punishment but as a positive method of teaching the child that he needs a time-out to reorganize himself.

  - Requesting a time-out is a constructive method of taking a break when the child is on sensory overload, is anxious, or has a self-regulatory disorder. Teach the child to request a break to reorganize constructively.

  - An adult time-out is a technique to interrupt attention-seeking behaviors and to reward appropriate behavior. The adult stops and shuts down all work, averts his eye gaze for fifteen or twenty seconds or until the child's behavior quiets or becomes appropriate, and then rewards the next appropriate behavior.

Handling Temper Tantrums and Challenging Behaviors

9

Temper tantrums are uncontrolled expressions of anger that consist of verbal and physical outbursts. They are attention-getting behaviors that occur when the child is feeling frustrated or angry and has no other way to address physical or emotional challenges of the moment. His emotions are stronger than his ability to control them. Tantrums are considered a normal part of development in children ages one to three because they lack the needed self-control, become easily overwhelmed by their emotions, and have limited coping strategies.

Typical characteristics of a tantrum include crying, whining, screaming and shouting, tensing the body, arching back or flailing arms, and throwing the body onto the floor. They normally last approximately two minutes, with the first thirty seconds being the most intense. Tantrums that are longer or more aggressive are not typical and include behaviors such as kicking, biting, hitting, scratching, pinching, pulling hair, throwing or breaking things, breath holding, or head banging. More aggressive tantrums are discussed at the end of the chapter.

Tantrums: Eighteen Months to Three Years

During the child's first twelve months of life an adult takes care of his every need. He is fed, bathed, cared for, and entertained. By having his needs met twenty-four hours a day, he is learning valuable lessons about trust and love and is developing strong emotional bonds with his parents. Somewhere around twelve to eighteen months the parents start to back off, no longer meeting his every need. The child is physically capable of doing things for himself and the parents' expectations change. Instead of doing for the child twenty-four hours a day, the parent allows the child more freedom and independence, encouraging the child to actively do things for himself. With this comes rules, limitations, and the word *no*. While the child actively embraces this new sense of freedom, independence, and opportunity to master new skills, there are times when the past (expectation to be cared for) and the present (drive for independence) collide. The child is new to this world with only one to two years of experience, his personality is barely developed, and he has very little self-control, tolerance for delayed gratification, or self-discipline. In addition, the two-year-old has a vocabulary of only about fifty words. His sentences consist of two words. With luck the adult understands about fifty percent of what the child is trying to communicate. He expects the world to respond to him as it has for the first year of life; he expects to get everything he wants, and when it doesn't happen he temporarily goes crazy in a fit of rage, overwhelmed by his emotions. He gets angry when he is not allowed to be independent or when he cannot figure out how to master a new skill, such as pouring a glass of milk or putting on his shoes. The clash between the child wanting to be independent, and not being physically or emotionally developed enough, may lead to strong emotions of anger and frustration. He does not have the coping skills or the tolerance to deal with the strong emotion and utilizes the only way possible to vent his frustration—he explodes into a tantrum.

Tantrums may be caused by several factors:

- Frustration with the world
  - Unable to complete a task independently (skill mastery)
  - Unable to communicate what he wants
  - To obtain something—object, activity, or event
  - To avoid something—task, activity, event, or person
- Feeling hunger
- Being tired
- Feeling uncomfortable
- Needing to seek attention; negative attention from a tantrum is often better than no attention

Tantrums are a natural stage of development for two-year-olds as they learn they can't have everything they want and can't always do something themselves, creating a power struggle with the adult. A child's temperament or family stress can make him vulnerable to tantrums. The child who is overly sensitive, overreacts to pain, or is quick to over-stimulate is more likely to overreact to road blocks in his autonomy and mastery of tasks. Personal or family stress: living in cramped quarters or in family situations that may include fighting, violence, emotional difficulties, alcohol or drug use, may make the child more susceptible to tantrums.

Tantrums will often continue through the third year of life, disappearing by the age of four when children develop the necessary motor and physical skills to be self-reliant. Their language skills have grown sufficiently to express their anger, solve problems, and compromise. They have developed the needed self-control and coping strategies to avoid tantrums. Nevertheless, some preschoolers and kindergarteners will still throw a tantrum if they have learned that a temper tantrum is a good way to get what they want.

Tantrums that occur in children over the age of four or in children with atypical development should be taken very seriously. The development of self-control and coping strategies may be more difficult to attain when there are underlying problems causing the tantrum.

Avoiding Tantrums

A toddler is young and vulnerable. His strong-willed and persistent behavior is characterized by immaturity. His outbursts are due to his inability to cope with his emotions. We need to set him up to succeed, not to be vulnerable. To do this we need to think in advance and plan ahead, know when the child is more likely to throw a tantrum, and try to avoid it. Here are some strategies to help avoid tantrums:

- Help the child develop good communication skills. Encourage the child to use his words to make his needs known and to describe his feelings. Teach him to ask for help and to label his emotions, such as "I'm sad" or "I'm angry."

- Teach the child to express anger constructively.

- Help the child develop strategies to calm himself down when he is getting excited. Identify calming activities such as drawing, playing with a favorite toy, or listening to music.

- Make sure the child is not tired or hungry.

  - Teach him to recognize when he is tired or hungry.

  - Teach him to label those feelings and to deal with the problem in constructive ways.

- Allow transition time when changing activities. Give a five-minute notice when changing from a desirable task to something less desirable, for example, coming in from outside and going to dinner or bed.

- Prepare the child for new situations or new people. Explain beforehand what to expect when visiting a new place, establish rules, and review them. For example, prepare the child for crowds or noise at a shopping center, and tell him he will need to hold your hand.

- Provide activities at the child's developmental level.

- Give positive attention to on-task behavior. Praise the behavior, whether the child is successful at the task or not. Avoid frustration and boredom.

- Give the child choices. Whenever possible do not give "no" answers—give alternatives instead. Do not say, "You can't have the ice cream." Instead give a choice: "You can have this orange or apple juice."

- Give the child control over little things to fulfill his need for independence. For example, "Do you want to sit at the table before or after you jump on the trampoline?" or "Do you want apple juice or orange juice?"

- Never ask a question when there is no choice. For example: "Do you want to eat?" or "Do you want to go to therapy?"

- Avoid power struggles. Find a compromise. Instead of the adult's way or the child's way, find an alternative. Whenever possible have the child come up with the idea.

- Choose your battles. When the child communicates he wants something consider the request carefully.

- Keep off-limit objects out of sight and out of reach of the child.

- Distract the child from the off-limit object. Take advantage of his short attention span.

  - Begin a new activity.

  - Replace the desired object with an allowed toy.

  - Change the environment.

- Stick to routines.

- Let the child know the rules and stick to them. Everyone involved with the child must know the rules and stick to them.

- Recognize the warning signs and try to intervene before the tantrum. Before the child is out of control, get down to the child's eye level and tell him he is getting too excited and needs to slow down, and then give him several choices of activities.

Whenever possible, emotionally help the child avoid a tantrum. Teach him that he is starting to escalate and help him regain composure. Get eye level with the child; hold him gently but firmly by the shoulders until you have eye contact; then speak to him. That way, your message is likely to be heard. If that doesn't work, distract him. Having a child go over the edge into a tantrum is not pleasant for anyone; help the child before it happens.

Handling a Temper Tantrum

When a child begins to throw a tantrum, the first thing to remember is: *Do not react. Remain calm!* Reactions involve emotions, which tend to reinforce the behavior. Toddlers are not able to handle their emotions, are trying to learn who they are, and do not have the coping skills to handle these situations. Do not complicate this emotionally charged experience with your own frustrations. If your emotional tone increases, so will the child's, and the tantrum will become exaggerated. By remaining calm, you can control every aspect of your response. Respond as if the behavior were not occurring. Your voice must not change inflections or rise in volume. Avoid even the smallest change in body language and facial expression. Do not escalate with the child; breath deeply and slowly.

Protect yourself, others in the area, and the child from harm. Maintain a calm, controlled affect. Assess the environment to assure that no one will be hurt. Unobtrusively move dangerous objects from the area without attending to the child's behavior. Be prepared to quietly step out of the way of flying arms and legs. Safety must be a top priority. Be firm and inflexible if the child starts resorting to behaviors that are harmful to others, such as throwing objects or hitting. Let him know that hitting is not an acceptable expression of anger. Hold him firmly by the shoulders and tell him to take deep breaths. If he says he cannot, do it with him. The goal is to get him to take the deep breaths next time before he starts hitting or throwing things.

Ignore the behavior unless the child is harming himself or others. Do not say "no!" Do not try to stop the tantrum in the middle or try to rationalize with him, as that often makes it worse. Logical explanations are unlikely to be heard through the crying and yelling. Do not change your "no" to a "yes" just to get the child quiet. Do not address the behavior verbally or look at the child. Children are sensitive to the smallest changes and will pick up on the subtlest cue that you have responded. Turn to help another child or walk away from the child while he is screaming (secretly making sure he is safe). If he follows you screaming or crying, pick up a book or magazine, or go into another room. While going into another room may have a powerful effect upon the child, remember he is having difficulties handling his emotions (usually anger or frustration), and dealing with abandonment issues on top of that may be more than he can handle. Choose your strategies based on the child's needs and developmental level. Acknowledging the child's feelings without reinforcing the tantrum or giving in to him can be done by simply saying, "Wow! You're really mad. Let me know when you are done." Then, walk away. Why ignore a tantrum? First, a child throwing a tantrum has mentally and physically lost it. You cannot reason with him when he is in this state, so do not try. Second, giving children attention when they have lost all behavioral and emotional control will inspire them to continue. The more you try to convince them to stop, the more rewarding the experience. The reward of negative attention during and after a tantrum feeds into children's love of attention and is a strong reinforcer.

Do not bribe a child to stop a tantrum. When you try to bribe him, you not only draw attention to the tantrum, thereby reinforcing it, but also teach the child that if he acts inappropriately he will be rewarded. Do not punish a child by hitting or spanking him. It draws strong negative attention to the tantrum, reinforcing it, and teaches the child that physical force is okay. It also teaches the child to avoid the adult when he is confused, doesn't know what to do, and is most in need of an adult to help him. Instead, move away from the child when he displays negative behaviors or tantrums and move toward him when he calms and shows positive behaviors.

Time-outs can be effectively used to avert a tantrum and to assist the child in calming down afterwards (see chapter 8, Behavioral Intervention Techniques).

Some children need help calming down, thereby not allowing you to move away from them. A child may frighten himself at the strength of his outburst and find that he does not know how to put an end to it. Once escalated, he cannot break the cycle without assistance. Some strategies that work include:

- *Pick him up and hold him firmly,* stopping the arms and legs from flailing. This will give him a sense of self, and therefore, control.

- *Take him out of the situation.* Move to a new environment, give him space to calm down and get some air.

- *Slowly count to 100 while holding him firmly.* Repetitive counting is calming. If you can engage the child in counting it will calm him faster. Loosen your hold on him as he calms.

- *Hold him firmly and hide his face.* If you cannot change environments, make him feel like he is by covering his face. It will help him calm and regroup.

During the tantrum phase, you should move away from the child, unless he needs help calming down. As the child calms, move towards him and praise him for calming down. Comfort him, but do not give into his demands. Respect his emotions while reinforcing his ability to calm down. Rules for this phase include:

- Do not make fun of the child or belittle him for his tantrum.

- Do not punish him. He may start to bottle up his anger, which could be unhealthy.

- Do not label the child a bad boy or girl.

- Do not give him a treat or reward him for calming.

Time the tantrum. It will make you feel good to know that ignoring the behavior is really working. Tantrums usually become worse after you first start to ignore them, as the child will work harder to get your attention. Then they will decrease over the following weeks as the child learns that the behaviors do not work for him and as he learns to tolerate his frustrations.

After the Tantrum Resolves

After the tantrum resolves most children are vulnerable. They were less than adorable, completely lost control of their behaviors and emotions, and now need reassurance that they are loved. Our response must be that we love them no matter what, but we did not like how they expressed their need, want, or emotions. The goal is to teach better ways to communicate, express, and handle their emotions so they do not need to throw tantrums.

Analyze the situation—what actually happened. Because we are dealing with toddlers with rudimentary reasoning skills and a low capacity to handle strong emotions, the analysis may be easy, but it is critical. How we deal with the child when he comes down from the tantrum is determined by what caused it. Did he experience a disappointment? Did he want a toy he couldn't have? Was he frustrated he couldn't get his shoes on by himself? Was he mad because you wouldn't let him stay up late?

Once the child is calm, acknowledge his feelings. For example: " I know you were frustrated that you couldn't get your shoes on" or "I know you wanted that toy and you were angry you couldn't have it." Talk with him about his frustrations and try to solve the problem, if possible. Explain to the child that there are better ways to get what he wants and teach him these strategies: "When you use your words, I understand. When you cry and scream, I don't." You must convey to him that when he uses his words and remains calm you will listen, and that tantrum behavior will not get your attention. Teach the child constructive outlets for his emotions. Be a good role model and teach him how you handle anger and frustration. The next time a similar situation arises, intervene before the temper tantrum. Offer assistance, give a choice, or anticipate the reason for the child's frustration and work to avoid it and the tantrum.

More Aggressive Tantrums and Behaviors

Tantrums are traumatic and are always taken seriously, but certain situations require special attention. The toddler who has atypical development may not grow out of this phase without special assistance. Speech delays and fine or gross motor difficulties make a child vulnerable to continue using tantrums beyond three years of age. All of the strategies discussed in the preceding section for the younger child apply to the child who is older or has atypical development. The older child may use tantrums for similar reasons as the toddler, he may not have the communication skills or cannot cope with frustration and anger, but now more complex reasons surface. It may be a learned response, a coping strategy, or a sensory issue that was not recognized when he was younger. The tantrums may be more aggressive than other children's and include kicking, biting, hitting, scratching, pinching, pulling their hair, throwing or breaking things, breath holding, or head banging. These are high-risk behaviors that are priorities for change.

Avoid the Tantrum

It is important to focus efforts on avoiding the temper tantrum. Children display warning signs before a meltdown. Often these may include nail biting, flushing of the face or body, grinding of teeth, fidgeting, whining, and/or tensing of muscles. This is the time to recognize the warning signs and begin analyzing their cause. This is your chance to intervene and avert the impending crisis. It is also the opportunity to teach coping skills and self-awareness to many children.

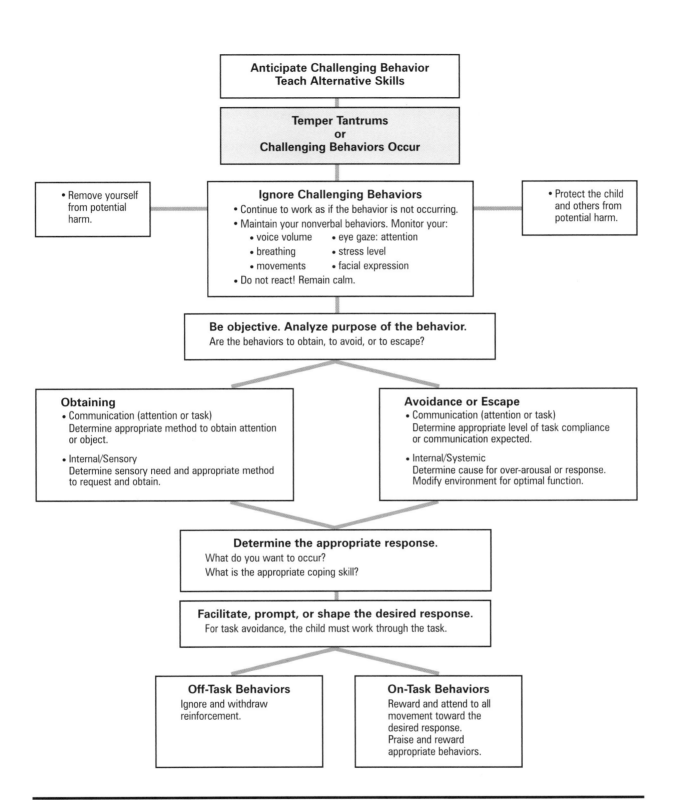

Figure 9.1   Handling temper tantrums and challenging behaviors

Based on your analysis of the cause you have several options:

- *Use Sensory-Based Activities*

  - The child is about to tantrum (lose his self-regulation). Consider sensory-based activities or repetitive, rhythmic activities for self-regulation before the tantrum. You may use heavy work or resistive activities to take advantage of the calming influences of proprioceptive input.

  - Sensory-based activities applied before a temper tantrum do not reinforce the tantrum but may aid in averting one. Do not use sensory-based activities that the child perceives as enjoyable after an outburst or tantrum. This will reinforce the tantrum.

  - Sensory-based activities can be used to increase the appeal of the activity or to provide a calming influence. You might give the child the choice of performing the task or doing a harder sensory-based activity. Make sure that the sensory-based activity will help calm and regulate him.

- *Intervene for obtaining behaviors.* Refer to appendix E, Intervention for Challenging Behaviors/Obtain, under Intervention.

- *Intervene for avoiding behaviors.* Refer to appendix E, Intervention for Challenging Behaviors/Avoid, under Intervention.

- *Use strategies discussed in this chapter under* "Avoiding Temper Tantrums."

Vivian starts to escalate as she is asked to begin a writing task. In order to avert a tantrum she is asked, "Do you want to do writing or do you want to do push-ups?" Vivian chooses to do push-ups. After a vigorous workout, Vivian is given a choice between writing or performing another set of push-ups. She chooses the push-ups again. After the third request, Vivian happily chooses writing. The heavy work calmed, organized, and focused her so she could cope with her anxieties over writing.

Everyone can use a break once in awhile. Is this what the child needs to avert the crisis? Carefully weigh whether you allow the child to leave the task for any reason. Letting the child up to move around signals that the task you are involved in is over. Getting him back to task will likely trigger a tantrum.

Proceed cautiously. Whenever possible, work the child through the issue, teaching him to work outside of his comfort zone without exploding. In some cases the child may not be able to do this without being given an opportunity to first calm himself. This may be done by removing him from the environment, using a time-out or distracting him.

Handling the Tantrum

Once the rage of a tantrum has started, the basic principles for handling a tantrum hold true: Stay calm and ignore the negative behavior. However, in older children and those with atypical development it becomes more complicated. The tantrums may be more aggressive, the behavior more difficult to analyze, and our emotions more complex.

A child may test you to see how far he can push you or find out whether you really mean what you say. He may throw himself on the floor screaming, bang his head, kick, scratch, lunge at you, bite either himself or you, throw things, and lash out at you verbally or physically. You will need to make decisions and take action immediately to deal with these behaviors. Knowing the most productive thing to do challenges even the most experienced professionals.

A child lunges at you, kicks and strikes out at you. You try to hold her to calm her and she bites you. Your automatic instinct is self-protection and anger. Your heart rate escalates and your body prepares for a fight. These are strong emotions that will interfere with handling the behavior objectively.

The first thing to remember is **do not react!** This may be easy when looking at a small toddler trying to assert himself, but becomes much harder with an older child who you think should know better. Our first reaction may be to fight back when we are attacked, avoid situations that are frightening and unpleasant, to blame someone when something goes wrong, or to comfort a child who is crying. Reactions rely on instinct, and our first instincts or impulses are usually counterproductive to the situations. Reactions involve emotions, which tend to reinforce the behavior and penalize the child with our judgments.

We must not personalize the experience. All too often we charge these behaviors with emotions and personalize the experience, especially when we are dealing with older children. Often statements arise that reveal we blame the child for willful behavior: "He hurt me," "That child is mean," "She's spoiled," or "Someone needs to teach her a lesson." These feelings and thoughts must be controlled. They reflect a conclusion based upon a lack of knowledge about the child, the child's behaviors, and what the child is trying to accomplish. These types of conclusions will block your ability to find the root of the problem and handle the child's behaviors constructively. You must control your thoughts in order to control your feelings and emotions. You must realize that the child is not maliciously attempting to hurt you. Tantrums are the only way the child knows of expressing stress and coping with problems and other emotions to which he sees no other solution. He has learned to use this behavior to cope.

The steps in effectively handling tantrums include: (1) remain calm, (2) ignore the behavior, and (3) protect *yourself, others, and the child from harm*. With more aggressive tantrums this becomes more difficult. Ideally, you should unobtrusively move dangerous objects from the area without attending to the child's behavior and quietly step out of the way of flying arms and legs. However, you might find yourself in need of physically protecting the child from harm, holding him firmly to protect him and you from danger. As he calms down you may keep your hands gently on the child so that you can feel changed muscle tone that may indicate a sudden advance toward you.

Challenging behaviors (hitting, biting, kicking, and more) can be seen in a full tantrum or as isolated behaviors. The procedure for handling a challenging behavior is the same. In some cases, where the child has not had a complete meltdown, you can continue working with the child while he engages in his negative behaviors. Ignore and do not react to the negative behaviors as you facilitate the child through the task or situation, working with the child to increase his tolerance.

Analyze, for the future, what you would have liked the child to have done instead of escalate. Facilitate that response the next time the child is in the situation.

Analyze the situation. Review the sequence of events and the probable causes for the behavior. What just happened? What is the child attempting to tell you? Does he want something (obtaining behavior), or is he avoiding something? Use the graphs and charts provided (handling temper tantrums, Figure 9.1, analyzing sensory behaviors and analyzing non-sensory behaviors, appendix D) to understand the exact cause for the behavior. Remember that many of the tantrum behaviors such as head banging, biting, throwing oneself on the floor, hitting, and pinching, provide intense sensory input (refer to appendix C), and may be a primary reinforcer to the tantrum. Therefore, a course of action that involves only ignoring the behavior will not be effective.

Determine a constructive course of action. What do you need to have happen, or what do you want the child to learn from this episode? The answer will be based upon your analysis of what triggered the behavior and what the child is trying to obtain or avoid.

There are some basic rules when determining an intervention program and avoiding secondary reinforcement to the challenging behaviors.

- Reward all constructive and positive behaviors. Reward them immediately and frequently.

- The instant disruptive behaviors occur, avert your eyes in order not to reinforce the behavior. Discontinue any positive praise.

- Prompt desired positive responses and shape appropriate responses. Reward all attempts in the correct direction.

- If the child is using a behavior to avoid a task, do not permit him to succeed. Ignore the behavior and work through the task. Be sure that the task is appropriate for the child. If necessary, modify the task for fewer repetitions. Be sure the child knows how many more repetitions are expected.

- If the child's tantrum behavior provides sensory input that is reinforcing or rewarding to the child, then ignoring the behavior will not be enough. Intervention must involve addressing the sensory need and behavioral strategies to extinguish the negative behavior. (Refer to Nonproductive Sensory-Obtaining Behaviors in chapter 5 and Behavioral Intervention Techniques in chapter 8.)

- A child may need to be removed from the situation or calmed if he is unable to regain his composure. The child may be so disorganized, upset, and anxious in the situation that he may need to be removed in order to calm himself.

  - Sensory-based activities or repetitive, rhythmic activities for self-regulation may be used to calm him. Examples might include deep breathing or slow counting.

  - Distracting him from the anxiety-provoking activity also may be effective. Engage him in a distracting task, and reward him for appropriate responses and on-task behavior.

  - Once calmed, place him back in the original situation that he attempted to avoid. If the child succeeds in avoiding the original task, the negative behavior will be reinforced and will continue.

  - The goal is not to complete the task, but to re-engage the child in the task and to end the task on a positive note.

Jasmine is asked by her teacher to write her first and last name. She begins to cry. When pressed to perform the task, her behavior escalates. She begins to scream and strike out at the teacher, hitting and kicking her. Without emotion or eye contact, the teacher turns her around in her seat and asks her to take deep breaths, coaching her and praising her efforts. Once calmed, she is turned back around to face the writing task and given the instruction, "Let's write your name together." The teacher prompts her through the task, one letter at a time, offering assistance as needed. Jasmine is then rewarded for task performance by allowing her to get out of her seat to read a book for three minutes.

The rules were followed here. The desired behavioral response was for Jasmine to cooperate in writing her name. Her crying, screaming, and aggressive behaviors were ignored and eye contact removed when the teacher turned Jasmine around in her seat. The teacher assisted in calming Jasmine by prompting deep breathing techniques, physically assisting Jasmine during the task, and rewarding Jasmine for her accomplishment. Her tantrum was not rewarded, as Jasmine was unsuccessful in avoiding the task.

A child lunges at you and starts to kick and hit because you brought out a new project for him to work on. You calmly step aside, and the child's lunge misses you. The child is in an open area and can't get hurt. You attend to another child in the area calmly, rewarding that child for good behavior, and ignore the child tantruming while remaining out of his reach. When he calms down you escort him to his seat and engage him in the new activity, praising his good behavior.

A child bursts out in tears, throws herself on the floor crying uncontrollably. You analyze the situation and realize that she is trying to avoid the task you brought out for her to do. You analyze the appropriateness of the task and know it is at her level. You bring her to the chair and begin to work with her, hand-over-hand, to have her complete the task. She tries to throw herself backwards, but you calmly continue. She quiets for one second, you praise her good work, and continue to work with her.

A child starts screaming and tries to run away. You try to guide her back, and she screams louder. Nothing you do quiets her; she continues to escalate, screaming and now fighting. There's no logic to it. You assess the situation and regain your composure. You are still unsure of what is triggering the behavior. Is it sensory modulation? Is it an expression of a want or need? It doesn't seem like task avoidance—she normally likes the activity. You lower your voice, slow your breathing, and watch for a moment. You take her hand and guide her from the area, reassuring her that you want to understand and help her. You engage her in a familiar activity, physically prompting her to complete the activity, obsessively counting out loud each repetition. She starts to count with you. She calms down and you return to the original room. You work on resistive activities that help her organize herself further, and then present the original task. She quietly completes the activity.

Working through the tantrum by removing her from the environment, engaging her in a familiar task, repetitively counting, and using resistive tasks helps her regain her self-control and self-regulation. Returning her to the original room and task eliminates rewarding the behavior by avoiding the task.

Consistency is critical when responding to challenging behaviors. Each professional must address the challenging behavior in the same manner in order to extinguish it. Once the behavior is exhibited, it must be addressed calmly and systematically. Secondary reinforcers, such as attending to the behavior, will cause the behavior to persist.

Anticipating the Challenging Behavior

A word of caution: Choose your battles wisely. Children respond for very specific reasons. These reasons can be predicted and anticipated. Know the child, read the warning signs, anticipate the behaviors, and avert crisis when possible.

Anticipating the child's behaviors is the most effective method of teaching coping skills. Keep alert for the signals that the behavior is about to occur, intercede as you start to see the signs, and teach the child alternative methods of responding. Do not allow yourself to be distracted by others in your environment. When you let your guard down, you will miss the warning signs and most likely will experience a disruptive behavior that could have been redirected. Learn from each experience, and whether teaching coping skills or handling a behavior, always try to end on a positive note.

Working Together as a Team

Parents often invest extensive time and energy in attempting to understand and explain their children's behaviors and intentions. This is exhausting and time consuming. It requires sensitivity to the multiple causes in the children's environments and within their bodies, as well as a keen sensitivity to the children themselves. Parents are invested in their children, and in some regards, overly sensitive to their needs, behaviors, and wants. Those children rely on the parents to meet their every need. While driven by love, and a need to do the best for their children, it is often hard for them to be objective regarding their behaviors and causes. As the children grow older, secondary rewards become more complicated and the causes are often not limited to a single factor. Parents often need and seek out the help of professionals who will respect their opinions as full, vested members of the team and will share their love and compassion for their children.

Professionals have a responsibility to assist the parents. They must respect the opinions of the parents as team members who have valuable insights into the child and how the child functions across multiple environments. The parents also often possess an innate sense of their children. It is the professional's responsibility to help the parents examine such information objectively and provide in-depth insights into their children.

Each specialist must assist in the development of effective remediation strategies and coping skills. This requires a comprehensive team approach between the behavioralist, occupational therapist, speech and language pathologist, physical therapist, special education instructor, augmentative communication specialist, parent, and physician. Working together, they develop and implement a comprehensive intervention program. Such a program is aimed at eliminating challenging or disruptive behaviors that interfere with the mastery of new skills, remediating the original underlying problem that causes the behavior and providing emotional support and encouragement.

Collecting data, identifying and analyzing problems, and developing an intervention program must be objective in nature. However, the success of an intervention program is often contingent upon the relationship between the professional and the child. In implementing the intervention program, the professional working with the child must *like* the child. Each child possesses strengths along with weaknesses, and anyone who expects to be effective in working directly with the child must be able to see the child's positive aspects.

Just as parents have an innate sense about their children, children have an innate sense about people around them. They can sense when a professional is afraid of them, appalled at their behavior, or just does not like them. Love and compassion toward another human being is projected through verbal and nonverbal behaviors. Inherent in this relationship are mutual trust and respect. To effectively change behaviors, we must not only provide emotional support and encouragement, we must also like the child (Murray-Slutsky and Paris 2000).

Summary

Tantrums are to be expected in the range of eighteen months to three years of age. They are developmentally appropriate and must be dealt with.

Tantrums occurring in children under eighteen months old, over the age of four, or in children with atypical development should be taken very seriously.

Challenging behaviors may be seen as part of a tantrum (complete physical and emotional breakdown) or in isolation. Intervention is similar to that of a tantrum.

Tantrums are windows of opportunity to establish and develop:

- methods of communication between the child and adults.

- self-regulation and emotional control.

- appropriate environmental interactions.

Avoid the tantrum through:

- Addressing the child's basic needs.

  - Environmental modifications (task structure, environment, personal style and approach) to lessen the likelihood of tantrums (see chapter 7, Environmental Intervention Techniques)

  - Assisting in self-regulation

  - Meeting the child's internal systemic needs (e.g., hunger, sleep)

  - Providing necessary sensory environment and activities for self-regulation

- Recognizing the early warning signs and intervening before the tantrum occurs.

  - Use sensory-based activities to:

    – Obtain sensory regulation.

    – Increase appeal of activity.

    – Provide a calming influence.

  - Teach the child to work through the episode, which may include temporarily removing him from the environment (time-out) or distracting him, if necessary.

  - Determine whether the behavior is for obtaining or avoiding and use the interventions outlined in chapters 5 and 6 and appendix E.

Handling a tantrum involves remaining calm, ignoring the child's negative behaviors, and protecting yourself and others until the behaviors resolve. You must remember that this is the only way the child knows to express stress, cope with problems, and handle a host of other emotions. They see no other solution. Our job is to teach them new strategies.

Whenever possible, work the child through the activity or event while ignoring the negative behavior. Do not discuss the event or behavior at this time. Merely move the child through the task.

If you cannot move the child through the task, it is important that you (or anyone in the environment) do not pay attention to his behavior. If this cannot be done, you must remove him from the environment (time-out) until he can regain his composure.

Reward any constructive and positive behaviors immediately and consistently.

After he regains control, resume and complete the task, making any necessary modifications.

Many challenging behaviors (head banging, biting, hitting) provide sensory input that is rewarding to the child. Ignoring the behavior is not enough. Intervention must address the sensory needs and behavioral strategies to extinguish the negative behavior. (Refer to Nonproductive Sensory-Obtaining Behaviors in chapter 5 and Behavioral Intervention Techniques in chapter 8.)

End on a positive note. Learn from this tantrum. Acknowledge the child's feelings and encourage behaviors to help him cope the next time the situation arises: Use his words and constructive methods to deal with frustration and anger.

Sensory Diets **10**

Obtaining Normal Levels of Attention, Arousal, and Effort

Our goal is for the child to display the appropriate level of attention, arousal, and effort for the task at hand. For this to happen the child must register appropriate sensory information, adjust his arousal levels to be appropriate for the activity, and ignore irrelevant information. This occurs when the child is in the calm-alert state. *A calm-alert state is a window in which our ability to function is maximized.* It is a state in which we have a balance between the ability to attend to a stimulus or task and the level of arousal within our brains and bodies to prepare us to respond. When we are within this calm-alert state we have optimum sensory processing, registration, and arousal. We have sufficient levels of stimulation to be alert and to be able to attend, and we are open to learning, processing, functioning, and active participation, yet not to the point where stimulation begins to interfere with participation. Children with central processing disorders often have difficulty in attaining and maintaining the calm-alert state.

Self-regulation is the ability to attain, maintain, and change arousal levels appropriate for the task or situation. A child needs to change his arousal level to continually stay within the calm-alert state appropriate for each activity. This may involve increasing his arousal levels at some times of the day while decreasing them at others.

Some children have never experienced the calm-alert state appropriate for an activity. They either function in high gear or are sluggish, continually functioning in low gear. Children need to learn what it *feels* like to function in the calm-alert state. If a child has never known normal levels of arousal, he will never have a norm from which to judge future behaviors. Our goal is to have the child functioning at optimal arousal. This goal involves:

- Obtaining better modulation within the child's system through using sensory integrative treatment strategies.

- Teaching the child to seek out appropriate activities that meet his sensory and regulatory needs.

- Increasing his comfort and amount of time spent within the calm-alert state, appropriate for the activity.

Sensory diets become a key factor in obtaining self-regulation and altering the child's arousal levels to increase his ability to function. Sensory diets empower the child to modulate his own nervous system by selecting appropriate sensory-based activities and

---

This chapter is adapted with permission from Murray-Slutsky and Paris 2000.

learning strategies to stay within the calm-alert state. As the child adopts socially acceptable activities to meet his sensory needs, he no longer needs the less desirable and challenging behaviors, so they may be extinguished.

Sensory Diets

The term *sensory diet* was coined by Wilbarger (1984) and Wilbarger and Wilbarger (1991) to describe the principles related to sensory processing theory. A nutritional diet was used as a metaphor to explain the key ideas about sensory diets. While nutritional diets involve three well-balanced meals a day and a snack, most people acknowledge that the study of nutritional diet planning involves special knowledge about many complex factors. A well-balanced diet requires the right amounts and combinations of foods to maintain the body's blood chemistries and sugar levels within normal range at all times. Similarly, sensory diets require the right combinations of sensory input to keep an optimal level of arousal at all times.

As snacks do, some sensory-based activities may change our mood or state of alertness for short periods of time, while others (similar to nutritious meals) have longer-lasting effects on behavior and performance. We can achieve and maintain optimal levels of arousal for performance by timing and carefully selecting our sensory-based activities. This is important for any person but especially important for those with a disruption in sensory experiences or a decreased ability to engage in activities (Wilbarger 1995).

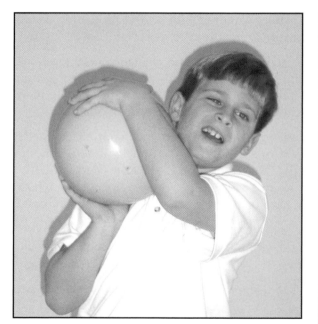

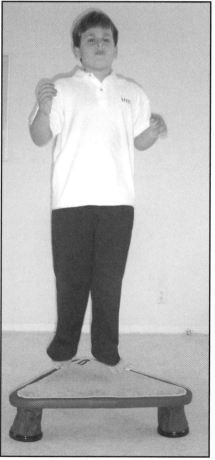

Weight lifting using the medicine ball and jumping on the bounce pad or trampoline have a modulating effect on the nervous system.

Certain types of activities have proven to have a modulating effect on the nervous system. Activities that include deep-touch pressure, vestibular, or proprioceptive inputs are believed to have the most pervasive effect on behavior. Examples include aerobics, weight lifting, jumping on a trampoline, play wrestling, or playing hard on playground equipment.

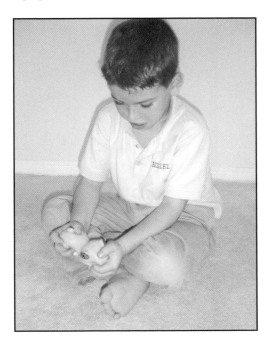

Fidgets, such as the Girgle Head Frog™, last only a matter of minutes but can help the child cope with changing needs or everyday stress.

Some of the most important changes in the nervous system come from knowing how to choose activities for long-lasting effects.

■ Specific vestibular activities such as vigorous swinging and jumping on a trampoline can last in the nervous system for four to eight hours.

■ Proprioceptive activities involving whole body, joint traction or co-contraction, or heavy muscle action as typified in rock-wall climbing, push-ups, and push-pull games generally have a two-hour duration within the nervous system.

■ Other activities—like snacks—are mood changers: They have a shorter effect on the nervous system, usually lasting only a matter of minutes, or as long as the child is engaging in the activity. They can elicit emotional responses, meet changing needs, and help you cope with everyday situations. These activities include tactile, visual, auditory, olfactory, and oral and respiratory inputs (Oetter, Richter, and Frick 1995). Activities may include:

  ▪ Sucking on candies,

  ▪ Chewing gum,

  ▪ Fidgeting with toys, and

  ▪ Listening to music.

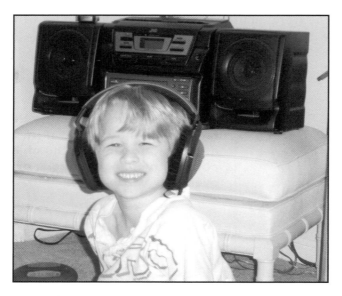

Listening to music or a Therapeutic Listening™ program can help children regulate and regain emotional and behavioral control.

By analyzing the child's sensory needs, daily routines, and arousal states throughout the day, an individualized sensory diet can be developed to optimize the child's performance, assuring that the child maintains the amount of arousal appropriate for functional tasks throughout the day.

Teach the Child Self-Regulation

The first step in developing a sensory diet is to analyze the child's sensory needs through a parent or teacher history form, interviews, and direct observation of the child. Questions and observations should revolve around:

1. The child's responses to experiences involving touch, tactile, or food choices, and his responses to vestibular or proprioceptive input, vision, auditory, smell, or taste.

2. Activities that are effective in calming, arousing, or organizing the child. It is often helpful to look at what sensory-based activities the child seeks or avoids, as well as the sensory components of any challenging or unusual behaviors displayed. Challenging behaviors develop initially to meet a sensory need, and then are maintained by the sensation they provide and the responses they elicit in the child's environment. Refer to appendix B for common behaviors observed, sensory input provided, and intervention strategies.

The next step is to analyze the child's arousal level and activity level throughout the day. Wilbarger (1995) recommends analyzing the sensory qualities encountered in two typical days: a structured school/work day and an unstructured day during the weekend. Record where the child sleeps, textures preferred in sheets and pajamas, his state when he gets up in the morning, and so on. Identify what part of the day the child is the most organized. During which part of the day is the child disorganized or is his behavior or performance diminished? Under what conditions does the child display low arousal levels versus high arousal levels? Are these predictable cycles?

Develop an Action Plan

Develop an action plan based on careful analysis of the child's likes, dislikes, and needs.

1. Identify the child's likes and needs (both are factors that contribute to the child's ability to function):

   ▨ Identify activities or sensory-based activities that are calming, pleasurable, and organizing for the child. Identify the activity, if it is socially acceptable. For activities that are not acceptable or desirable, identify the sensory component.

   ▨ Identify times and situations throughout the day in which the child functions optimally and operates in the calm-alert state. Define specific factors that appear to contribute to this state/behavior.

2. Identify negative factors, activities disliked or avoided, and activities that contribute to sensory overload or shutdown.

   ▨ Identify times and situations throughout the day in which the child does not function optimally. Define specific factors that contribute to this.

   ▨ Identify environmental factors that adversely impact the child's functional performance and contribute to sensory overload. Consider organizational aspects, sensory components, arousal levels, activity demands, and frustration levels created by the activity.

   ▨ Identify coping strategies that are either not effective or are not socially acceptable for the environment.

3. Establish an action plan.

   ▨ Identify several powerful sensory-based activities that are socially acceptable and effective in either raising or lowering the child's level of arousal into the calm-alert state. Determine the length of effectiveness of each activity.

   ▨ Establish therapeutic routines to increase the child's attention, organization, and arousal levels to optimize performance. Develop routines incorporating sensory-based activities that meet the child's arousal and organizational needs into all daily activities: waking up, dressing, and activities throughout school hours, during transitions, mealtime, leisure activities, bathing, bedtime, and so on.

   ▨ Modify the child's environment for optimal states of arousal and function.

   ▨ If necessary, teach the child to perform and use the sensory-based activity in order to derive the sensory experience and benefit from the activity.

   ▨ Teach the child self-regulation. Teach the child to identify signs of escalating behaviors or low arousal levels and to seek out appropriate sensory-based activities to help him obtain the arousal level appropriate for the activity.

The majority of children react in similar ways throughout the day. Their sensory registration, arousal, or attentional problem is characterized by either under- or overarousal to sensory information and is considered stable and predictable. The activities selected should address the individual child's arousal needs.

The Underaroused Child

Children who are underaroused often fail to register sensory information within the environment. They simply are unaware of people, things, and activities around them, so they do not or cannot interact with them. These children may resist participating in activities or perform activities poorly, have difficulty allocating attention to the activity or task, and may not assimilate information well. They often appear sluggish, withdrawn, tired, and uninterested. Underaroused children benefit from sensory-based activities that increase their overall arousal.

Sensory-based activities must be selected, tried, and monitored carefully for their effects on the child. Closely observe the child's reaction and facial expressions as you introduce new and more aggressive sensory input. You will be looking for an increased awareness, responsiveness, and processing of sensory information. It is important to remember that each child is different and that individual preferences, likes, and dislikes enter into designing the correct intervention that will bring the underaroused child into the window of the calm-alert state.

In general, linear vestibular movements in an up-down or forward-backwards direction, combined with deep-touch or proprioceptive input, have an arousing yet overall organizing effect on the nervous system. Activities that are repetitive, regular, and fast in nature will also have a more arousing yet organizing effect. In contrast, activities that are irregular in their speed, rhythm, or movement may have a disorganizing effect and should be avoided. Examples of fast, repetitive, regular activities that combine linear vestibular movements with deep-touch or proprioceptive input include:

- Jumping on a trampoline

- Riding a bicycle

- Jumping on a pogo stick

- Bouncing while sitting on a ball

- Jogging

- Using a scooter-board

- Linear swinging in the net or swinging in the net with the child propelling himself using a bungee cord

- Playing tug-of-war games

- Participating in extracurricular activities, such as karate, judo, Tae Kwon Do, horseback riding, bicycle riding, swimming, roller blading or skating, dancing, gymnastics, or other aerobic-type sports

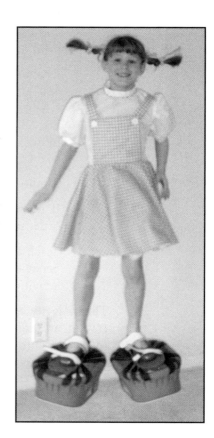

Moon Shoes™ provide linear vestibular input in combination with proprioception. Jumping activities provide fast repetitive and regular qualities needed for organizing the child.

When looking to increase a child's arousal, the entire therapeutic environment must be taken into consideration. Things to keep arousal levels increased include:

- A colorful, brightly lit room;

- Loud, high-energy instructions and interactions;

- Enthusiasm; and

- Verbalizations with inflections and changing pitches, gestures, and animation.

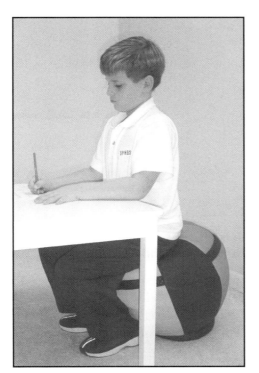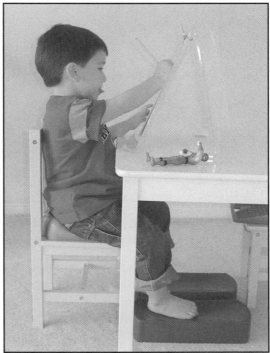

The Sit Ball™ and the Movin' Sit™ cushions provide vestibular input to the underaroused child, increasing his posture and arousal.

The Overaroused Child

In contrast, a child's nervous system may be overaroused. The child may be hyperresponsive, overregister to multiple stimuli, have difficulty filtering out pertinent from nonpertinent information, or not process information or assimilate it well. He may have difficulty in adapting to changes in his environment, have a level of arousal and attention that is not always appropriate, not block out irrelevant information, or attend to inappropriate things in his environment. Organizational problems, high anxiety levels, and low thresholds of frustration tolerances are inherent in an overaroused child. The child may have difficulty sitting still to complete a task; be unable to control his impulses; have difficulty monitoring and controlling his emotions, appearing as if he is about to blow up or lose control; or be in constant, yet nonproductive, motion.

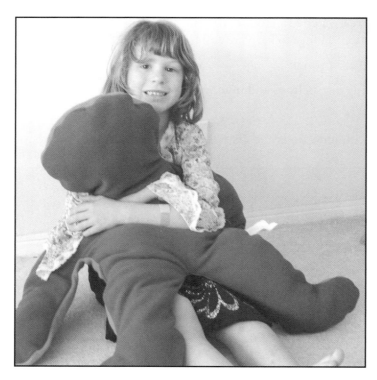

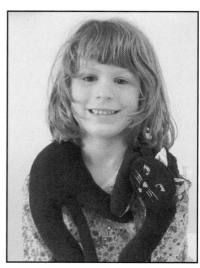

The Anybuddy™ provides deep-touch pressure and the Kitty Kuddles™ can be warmed. Both offer inhibition for the child who is overaroused.

Children who have difficulty handling multiple sensory stimuli within an environment, quickly become overaroused, or exhibit defensiveness, will benefit from inhibition techniques that are geared toward lowering their arousal level and anxiety. These techniques include modifying the environment and implementing systems that reduce anxiety. The goal is to move the child from overarousal to the calm-alert state in order to promote improved attention and task performance.

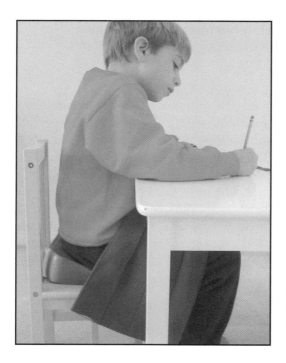

The weighted lap pad provides deep-touch input and helps the child relax into his chair.

Environmental factors play a major role in decreasing a child's arousal levels. Clutter-free environments, quiet enclosed rooms, predictable schedules, slow rhythms and songs, and low, monotone voices tend to be calming. Some children need to decrease environmental stimuli while receiving deep-touch input. These children benefit from having a hideout or quiet place to go to when they need to calm down and get organized. It can be a cardboard box with a top, a table placed in a corner with a blanket over it, or any small enclosure. Some children like to have pillows, foam blocks, or blankets placed in the box for deep-touch input.

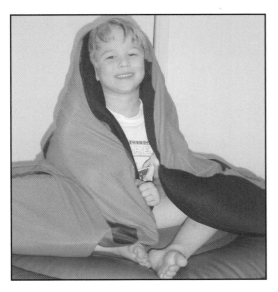 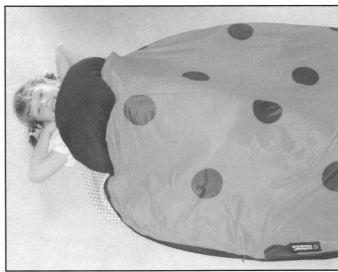

Children often seek the deep-touch and calming effect of weighted blankets.

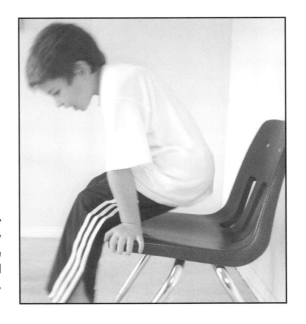

Push-ups done in a chair offer direct inhibition through heavy resistance and can easily be implemented in a school setting.

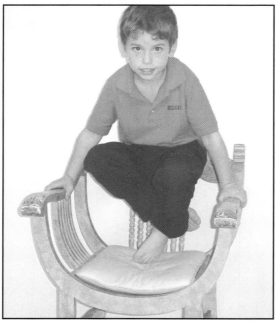

Chair push-ups can be done anywhere once taught.

Wall push-ups or hand-stands.

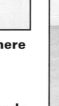

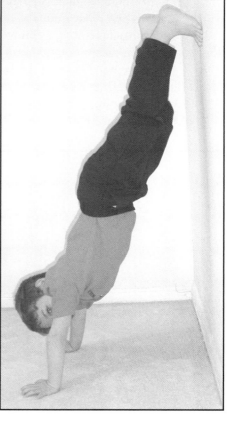

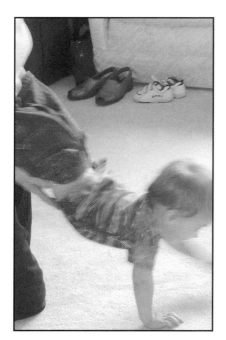

Wheelbarrow walks.

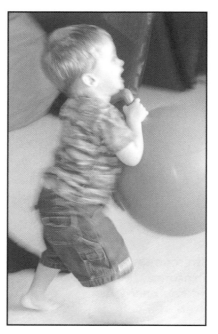

Carrying heavy objects or performing chores that require heavy work are calming activities.

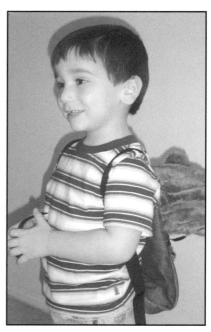

Backpacks or weighted backpacks provide proprioceptive input and are often used as part of a sensory diet.

Sensory-based activities to lower arousal levels need to include deep-touch input and proprioceptive input as well as environmental modifications. Deep-touch and proprioceptive activities are the most direct forms of inhibition, and therefore, are calming techniques that can last up to two hours. They include resistive activities, such as:

- Push-ups, performed against the floor or wall or between two desks (arm push-ups in which children lift their own body weight).

- Weight bearing on the arms (in which the child places his hands on the floor while supporting his knees on a chair). In this position, he may read or complete an activity.

- Wheelbarrow walks.

- Animal walks such as crab, bear, or duck walks.

- Isometric exercises such as pushing against an immovable object (e.g., a wall or clasping his hands together and pushing).

- Chores that require heavy work, such as moving furniture, carrying groceries, or pushing a cart filled with heavy supplies.

- Sports and extracurricular activities such as karate, Tae Kwon Do, judo, dancing, gymnastics, aerobic exercises, or sports. When choosing appropriate sports, look for activities that provide heavy work and strenuous exertion, without increasing defensiveness. For example, swimming has a tactile component, basketball and football have unexpected touch and vestibular input from being bumped. If the child reacts negatively to the sport or activity — respect his wishes.

It is important to identify the cause of the defensive behavior and the sensory systems involved. Intervention includes *taking out* factors that increase arousal and defensiveness while *putting in* sensory strategies to help calm and regulate the child, such as:

- Activities that incorporate deep-touch and deep-proprioceptive input and slow, rhythmic vestibular input work to inhibit and calm the nervous system.

- Inhibition techniques to decrease child's level of arousal (refer to appendix B).

- Environmental modifications to limit sensory overstimulation (see chapter 7, Environmental Intervention Techniques).

- Behavioral strategies to control impulsiveness and emotional responses and alter learned responses (see chapter 8, Behavioral Intervention Techniques).

- Avoid anxiety and threatening activities whenever possible, as they will block the child's ability to attend and process information.

Common defensive responses and suggested techniques that are often helpful for children with modulation disorders can be found in appendix B.

Fluctuating Arousal

It is normal for everyone to have fluctuating arousal levels throughout the day. Many people wake up in the morning underaroused. With the assistance of caffeine, exercise routines, or other morning rituals, they raise their arousal levels into the calm-alert state, ready to undertake the day. Arousal levels can change quickly, either increasing because of stress or daily challenges, or decreasing because of fatigue or boredom. Most adults can predict the points at which their arousal levels are outside the calm-alert state, and they make adjustments.

Fluctuating arousal levels that are predictable are more easily dealt with. When you can predict alterations in arousal levels you can anticipate the child's needs. A teacher knows that children need time to increase their arousal levels before study lessons; therefore, she schedules music or circle time with high-energy activities to increase arousal before the lesson. After lunch, arousal levels often dip, making this a perfect time to schedule play, nap, or art time. When you can predict arousal levels, you can strategically place activities that will either increase or decrease these levels throughout the child's day, thereby engineering the child into the calm-alert state.

Fluctuations in arousal become a problem when they are not predictable. It makes it difficult to plan activities or match the appropriate activity to the child's arousal level.

It is important to identify techniques to help the child function and stay in the calm-alert state. Activities geared toward increasing the child's arousal level should be used cautiously for a child with fluctuating arousal levels (modulation disorder).

- Use activities that incorporate deep-touch and deep-proprioceptive input and work to inhibit and calm the nervous system.

- Use inhibition techniques to decrease the child's level of arousal.

- Use facilitation techniques, cautiously, to increase arousal levels. When using vestibular input, use only linear combined with proprioception.

- Make environmental modifications to limit sensory overstimulation (refer to chapter 7, Environmental Intervention Techniques).

- Implement behavioral strategies to control impulsive, emotional responses and alter learned behaviors (see chapter 8, Behavioral Intervention Techniques).

- Avoid anxiety and threatening activities whenever possible, as they will block the child's ability to attend and process information.

- Fluctuating modulation disorders may be the result of an unstable and volatile nervous system or of an internal systemic problem and may require medical consultation. Activities geared at increasing the child's arousal level may contribute to the instability of the child's condition.

Table 10.1
Moving the Child Into the Calm-Alert State: Environmental and Therapeutic Modifications to Alter Arousal Levels

If Underaroused	If Overaroused
■ Use stronger modalities to increase arousal.	■ Use inhibition techniques.
■ Use fast, regular, repetitive type movement such as bouncing and jumping.	■ Lower anxiety: Use environmental and organizational modifications.
■ Use linear vestibular movement and deep-touch or proprioceptive input.	■ Use slow, rhythmic, repetitive activities, such as slow rocking.
■ Modify therapeutic environment with brightly lit rooms, bright colors, and fast rhythms and songs.	■ If it is calming, use deep-touch, deep-proprioceptive, and/or resistive input.
■ Modify therapeutic use of self. Use louder voice with changing inflections, high energy, enthusiasm, animation, and gestures.	■ Use neutral warmth or swaddling for young children.
■ Oral-motor activities, such as chewing and crunching, or flavors, such as sour, bitter, or hot, may be arousing.	■ Modify therapeutic environment: clutter free and organized; low natural lighting; quiet enclosed rooms; slow rhythmic songs.
	■ Modify therapeutic use of self. Use lower, softer, almost monotonous voice, and slow, calm speech. Avoid animation and exaggerated movements.
	■ Oral-motor activities, such as sucking or sweet flavors, may be calming.

Oral-Motor Activities: Related to Sensory Diets

Oral-motor activities have an impact on the tactile system. The mouth is reported to have more tactile nerve endings per square inch than anywhere else on the body. Tactile input has a direct impact on the arousal system within the body. What you choose to put in your mouth can either calm you or wake you up. We do this without thinking about it. If you're stressed, ice cream may be soothing; granola bars are crunchy and wake you up; sucking on peppermint candy can be relaxing; apples, carrots, or celery can help let out aggression and let go of stress; drinking from a sports water bottle can keep you focused.

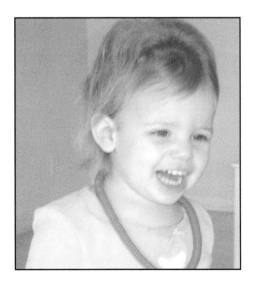

A chewy necklace provides her deep-proprioceptive input to help with self-regulation. It is available whenever she needs it.

The therapeutic value of oral-motor activities necessitates a more in-depth look. It is through coordinating suck, swallow, and breathing that the child starts to develop core stability. Slow, deep breathing, the cornerstone of many exercise programs, such as Pilates or yoga, is designed to increase core stability and to balance the body, mind and spirit. This core stability is believed to affect the child's emotional security and sense of self. The mouth and breath control are instrumental in developing core stability of the neck and trunk. Carefully choosing oral-motor activities can affect the child's arousal levels, self-regulation, his core stability, hand-eye control, and speech and language. The oral-motor activity you choose may depend on:

- The texture of the food item.

- What you do with the food item: bite it, suck it, chew it, drink it, lick it.

- The physical feeling of what you are doing as you chew, bite, or suck, which also involves the texture of the food or drink.

- The taste: sour, sweet, salty, spicy, or bitter.

- The temperature of the food, such as ice cream, hot chocolate, a cold popsicle, or warm soup.

- Tool usage: whistles, musical instruments, straws, sports water bottles.

- What you physically do with these items.

Tactile experiences of food in the mouth are the easiest, most natural way to give tactile stimulation and deep-touch input into the mouth and jaw. Look for snacks and foods that offer resistance and require the jaw and tongue to work hard. Teething biscuits are excellent methods for the young child to obtain both deep-touch and deep-proprioceptive input through biting. Chewy and crunchy foods, while requiring similar oral-motor control, have different impacts on the sensory system. Chewing is resistive and organizing, while crunchy foods are alerting. Chewy foods include bagels, gummy candies, cheese, gum, and granola bars. Crunchy foods that are alerting include popcorn, pretzels, bread sticks, crackers, fruit, nuts, and raw vegetables such as carrot or celery sticks.

Flavors and temperatures of candies and foods need to be taken into account and can be used to your advantage (Table 10.2). Sour foods, such as lemon, sour balls, or Mega Warheads®, are alerting, arousing, and organizing. Hot and spicy (cinnamon candies) or bitter flavors are even more alerting. For a child having difficulty attending or waking up, sour candies or a tablespoon of frozen lemon concentrate may do the job. A child who is oversensitive in the mouth may react better after using ice pops, ice cubes, or frozen juice cubes to desensitize the mouth. Cold temperatures of foods can be used to decrease sensitivity in most cases of oversensitivity and increase sensitivity in most cases of low tone and underarousal. When using ice to increase oral tone and oral movements the child should suck the ice for no more than one minute at a time. Take a one-minute break, then resume.

Table 10.2
Characteristics of Foods or Snacks

Chewing is resistive and organizing.	Chewy foods include: ■ Bagels ■ Gummy candies ■ Cheese ■ Gum ■ Granola bars
Crunching is alerting.	Crunchy foods include: ■ Popcorn ■ Pretzels ■ Bread sticks ■ Crackers ■ Fruit ■ Nuts ■ Raw vegetables, such as carrot or celery sticks
Sour foods are alerting, arousing, and organizing.	Sour foods include: ■ Lemon candies ■ Sour ball ■ Mega Warheads®
Hot, spicy, or bitter flavors are more alerting.	Hot, spicy, or bitter foods include: ■ Cinnamon candies ■ Atomic FireBall® candies
Cold food temperatures decrease sensitivity and increase low tone and arousal	

Just as we choose food to help alter our arousal levels, we use sucking, blowing, and biting to help us through difficult times in our day. We bite on our pencil or pen, chew our straw, chew gum, or drink from our water bottle. Suck, blow, bite, crunch, and lick are major components of oral-motor activity that can be incorporated into meals, snacks, and play activities with food or nonfood items. Use of these components along with taste, temperature, texture, size and form, and fit will work toward more functional synergy of suck/swallow/breathe elements. Blowing or sucking using whistles, straws, or musical instruments helps develop tongue, cheek, jaw and lip, and respiratory muscle control. Games can be developed combining flavors and temperatures with sucking and blowing activities, such as sucking Jell-O® through a straw or blowing bubbles using long tubing in a bottle of soapy water.

Oral-motor activities (eating, biting, crunching, blowing, or sucking) can help a child maintain self-regulation and the calm-alert state. They can help increase arousal in the morning, lower arousal levels at night, and maintain the calm-alert state during class time or homework activities.

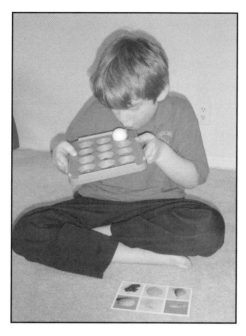

Blowing Lotto™ is a game that demands sustained blowing to help a child maintain self-regulation and the calm-alert state.

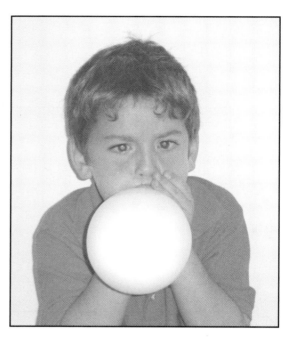

Blowing or sucking activities help develop tongue, cheek, and jaw and lip control as well as offer proprioception for self-regulation.

Setting Up a Sensory Diet

An occupational or physical therapist trained in sensory integration theory should develop sensory diets. Sensory strategies and therapeutic interventions are not usually skills the child automatically acquires. They must be selected for the individual, and the child must be taught how to perform them without injury. Moreover, the child often cannot perform therapeutically-based sensory activities initially without assistance. Use of novel activities, such as hideout or sensory boxes, may need to be introduced during therapy. Activities such as bike riding, push-ups, and so on, that the child is unfamiliar with may require training during therapy. The goals of therapy are to teach the child how to physically complete the activity, learn the organizing effects provided by the activity, and how and when to use the activity for self-regulation. Then we need to assist the family or teachers to gradually integrate the activities successfully into strategically placed intervals in the child's routine. It's important to note that when implementing sensory-based activities as part of a sensory diet, the activities should never be used as punishment but as a pleasant, organizing experience.

Children need to learn self-regulation. They are often unable to objectify or interpret their own behaviors, responses, or needs without assistance and guidance from an adult. We must help them understand and objectify what they are feeling or what they want. Once children can identify the need, they can be directed toward the activities that will meet the need. As they begin to recognize the signs that precede escalating behaviors and sensory needs, they will independently choose activities that help them maintain the calm-alert state throughout the day.

Sensory Integrative Treatments

Sensory integrative (SI) intervention is designed to address the underlying problems in sensory processing. SI interventions must be differentiated from sensory diets. Sensory diets, while addressing the sensory system, do no meet the essential characteristics of a sensory integration treatment. Sensory diets teach compensatory strategies that are effective in altering arousal levels and are based on sensory integrative principles. However, sensory diets are not the same as sensory integrative intervention.

The essential characteristics of sensory integrative intervention include:

1. The primary goals of SI therapy must aim at improving the underlying neurological process, rather than teaching a skill.

2. The child must be an active participant and activities should be primarily child-directed and intrinsically motivating.

3. The intervention is individualized to meet the developmental needs and goals of the client.

4. The activities must be purposeful, provide the "just-right challenge," and result in an adaptive response.

5. The activities provide enhanced sensory feedback with emphasis on tactile, proprioceptive, and vestibular systems.

(Ayres 1979; Kimball 1999; Koomar and Bundy 2002; Miller et al. 2002; Parham and Mailloux 2001)

Children who fit the picture of having a sensory integrative disorder or who need a sensory diet, often need sensory integrative intervention to address the underlying problems. They should receive an evaluation by a qualified occupational or physical therapist who has received postgraduate training in sensory integrative theory and treatment, or who has pursued certification or continuing education in this area. A therapist with the same qualifications should implement sensory integrative intervention.

Case Study: Adam's School Behavior

11

Adam, a seven-year-old, attends a regular second-grade class within a private school. He is a very bright child, and with his parents' help on his homework, is a B student. However, his behavior in class became a high priority for change, as he was about to be withdrawn from the school for disrupting his classroom.

When observed in the classroom, he exhibits out-of-seat behaviors, fidgeting, and other disruptions to the class. He rocks in his chair, puts his feet on the desk, and frequently falls out of his chair. He gets out of his seat, works standing, stands and supports his body weight on his hands, or stretches his arms and legs. He frequently knocks things off his or others' desks, bumps into children, and is disruptive to those around him. He appears inattentive and distractible.

There have been several parent-teacher conferences to report that his behavior is distracting to the teacher and other students and disrupts the classroom. His parents have taken away television and other privileges due to his "bad behavior" in school, but the behaviors have continued. The school psychologist has been consulted. Her recommendations consisted of behavioral strategies aimed at extinguishing the behavior by having the teacher attempt to ignore the behavior when it occurred or physically prompt him back to his seat. The teacher was advised not to reward the behavior with attention. Although the teacher admits that Adam manages to get most of his work done, she is frustrated at the constant classroom interruptions and cannot tolerate it any longer. In an attempt to avoid having him withdrawn from school, his mother decided to seek the aid of an occupational therapist with sensory integration (SI) specialization to help in analyzing Adam's behavior. The mother's question is, "Is it sensory or is it behavior?"

Let's follow the ABC's in analyzing the Behavior. Please refer to figure 4.1.

Step B: Identify and Define the Behavior.

Definition of behavior: Adam's behavior is identified as excessive body movements and out-of-seat behaviors that include, but are not limited to:

1. Rocking in his seat,

2. Putting his feet on the desk,

3. Stretching his arms and legs,

4. Falling out of his seat,

5. Standing at his desk, and

6. Standing, bearing his full body weight on his hands, as in arm push-ups.

Are the behaviors linked? Although the behaviors do not occur in a predictable sequence, they are linked because they may stem from a similar underlying cause yet to be determined.

Priority for change? The behaviors fall into the category of disruptive behavior and have a high priority for change because of the urgency of the school situation.

Step A: Look at the Antecedent

When does the behavior occur?

1. The behavior occurs only with seated activities in the classroom, library, or at home.

2. The behavior does not occur when he is seated watching television at home.

3. Specifically, he begins his school day with his head lying on the desk. When asked to sit up, his behavior grows increasingly restless until out-of-seat behaviors erupt.

4. Behaviors occur during teacher lecture, demonstration, and during written assignments.

In what environments does the behavior occur?

1. The behavior occurs as frequently in a one-to-one situation as it does in the classroom setting with thirty other children.

2. The behavior also occurs in small rooms as often as in the main classroom.

3. The behavior occurs when the classroom is quiet as well as when noise levels increase.

4. The environment, therefore, was not suspected as a primary cause.

What are the warning signs that the behavior is about to occur?

1. The teacher reported noticing a gradual increase in restlessness over the course of the morning.

2. She noted that Adam's distractibility increased rapidly when the class was asked to engage in a written activity or discussion.

Step C: What is the Primary Cause of the Behavior?

Is Adam doing his work? The answer to this question is that he is attempting to comply with all assignments but is struggling to get the work done. Therefore, we draw the conclusion that he is not seeking to avoid the work, so we believe he is seeking to *obtain* something.

Is he seeking to obtain a task or object? No.

Is he seeking to obtain attention? We must consider the responses of not only his teacher but also his peers to answer this question.

1. The teacher's response to the behaviors is to make repeated requests that single Adam out.

   ▪ "Put your feet on the floor," "sit up straight," "put your hands down if you don't have a question," "stay in your seat," and so on.

   Consider the frequency with which Adam is given one-on-one attention from the only adult in the room.

2. The response of Adam's classmates is to give him attention as well.

   - They laugh when he gets into "funny" postures, when he falls out of his seat, and when he frustrates the teacher.

   - Individuals react to him when he bumps into them, knocks items off their desks, or otherwise distracts them.

There is enough one-on-one attention directed toward Adam as a result of his behavior to warrant considering attention-seeking as a primary cause for his behavior. Let's continue the analysis.

Could the behavior be sensory-seeking for internal/systemic (sensory) reasons?

1. We recognize that the behaviors may serve to provide input from two sensory systems, namely the proprioceptive and the vestibular systems. All of Adam's out-of-seat behaviors are proprioceptive in nature, while his rocking and fidgeting behaviors are vestibular in nature.

2. We note that Adam begins his day lying on the desk. When asked to sit up and to work, his posture deteriorates over the course of the day, indicating a possible problem with postural control and endurance.

3. We know that hyposensitive or under-responsive children may seek vestibular and or proprioceptive input to stimulate or arouse their postural and attentional mechanisms. Adam's behaviors seem to fit into this explanation; therefore, sensory-seeking behaviors must be considered as a possible primary cause of the behaviors.

   Because Adam appears to be getting most of the work done, we must assume that the strategy *is productive* and works for him.

Could the behavior be avoidance behavior?

1. Task avoidance. Adam's behavior does not appear to be an attempt to avoid the tasks. On the contrary, he eagerly attempts to comply and complete the task. Although distractible, he struggles to participate in what is going on in the classroom.

2. Internal/Systemic avoidance. Adam does not appear overaroused or overwhelmed within the classroom. Internal/Systemic avoidance did not seem to apply to Adam's behavior and was therefore ruled out.

Intervention Plan

The intervention plan used a two-pronged approach that included intervention to remediate the underlying sensory integrative dysfunction while implementing behavioral strategies to make the behaviors less apt to occur.

By following the behavioral analysis graph located in appendix D, the occupational therapist designed a program for Adam.

Analyze the child's behavior and the activities the child engaged in to determine the sensory need being met.

1. What is/are the sensory system(s) that are under- or overresponsive?

   The occupational therapist found Adam to have low muscle tone and his behaviors to be characteristic of underresponsiveness to proprioceptive and vestibular inputs.

2. What is the sensory need the child is trying to accomplish when he engages in the activity?

Adam engaged in postures that increased the joint and muscle inputs through the stiffness levels of the muscles he used and through the bizarre postures he assumed, thereby increasing the proprioceptive input he received from his joints and muscles. He also derived vestibular input through the rocking of his chair and body, and as he moves from sit to stand and back to sit.

3. What does the behavior tell you about the sensory system?

Adam started each day with his head on his desk, a common occurrence in a child with low muscle tone and a tendency toward underresponsiveness. When asked to sustain an erect posture and attend to the classroom activities, his out-of-seat behaviors increased.

The conclusion to this analysis was that the *primary cause* of the behaviors was sensory in nature, and that Adam was *seeking* to increase his arousal level and his body awareness and to bolster his postural responses through proprioceptive and vestibular inputs. His rocking and out-of-seat behaviors were an attempt to self-regulate and modulate himself for classroom activities. Because the cause was sensory in nature, pure behavioral applications would not work in extinguishing the behaviors.

The fact that the behaviors worked for Adam was also a very strong primary reinforcer to the behaviors. By bolstering his arousal levels during times of the day and classroom activities in which his arousal level would normally plummet, the behaviors were ingrained as a strategy to be used whenever Adam felt the need to self-regulate.

4. What is the function served by the behavior if different from the sensory need?

Adam was not trying to avoid the task, but did get attention from his teacher and peers as a result of the behaviors. The *secondary reinforcers* were the attention from his teacher and the reactions of his fellow students. This was believed to be a consequence of the behaviors that served to reward Adam rather than serving as a primary cause for his behaviors.

Identify acceptable alternative sensory activities or behaviors that meet the same sensory need, at the same levels of intensity of sensory input and same duration and frequency.

Strategies here included the use of a wake-up exercise routine before school consisting of jumping on the mini trampoline. His sensory diet included an array of exercises interspersed throughout his day. He learned to do isometric and concentric exercises in his seat every hour. It took him an average of three to four minutes to complete his set of exercises. Thera-Band® was tied to the legs of the chair for resistive leg movements. He could push his legs against the stretchy elastic while staying seated. He also needed an inflatable cushion in his chair to help him keep his muscle tone up and not fall or move out of his chair. It provides additional vestibular input. The Movin' Sit™ cushion worked the best because its wedged shape kept him sitting upright, with his feet firmly planted on the ground. He was taught to request breaks to perform arm push-ups, chair push-ups, or hand-stands at the back of the room. The teacher began to realize he needed the exercise break almost every hour. Adam reported he had difficulty sitting quietly and waiting while the teacher organized work for the class. He liked the idea of using a fidget, a gel-filled ball on a key chain secured to Adam's belt. It kept his hands busy without disrupting others in the class.

For written activities, an incline board was recommended to lessen the postural demands placed upon him, to prevent the need for him to rest on the desk, to improve his visual attention to the task, and to aid him in monitoring his hands during writing tasks.

Address the underlying "function" served by the behavior.

The occupational therapy program was administered twice a week with goals to:

- Normalize his muscle tone,
- Improve his postural control,
- Improve grading of his movements,
- Improve his ability to perform slow sustained muscular efforts, and
- Teach him self-regulation strategies.

Treatment involved activities with enhanced vestibular and proprioceptive input. The therapist concentrated on teaching the skills needed for the recommended exercise program aimed at self-regulation (e.g., desk push-ups and hand-stands). She included strengthening of the muscles of the hand, wrist, and forearm, and activities to improve Adam's fine motor skills in order to make written work easier for him.

Use behavioral strategies to stop, alter, limit, or replace the behavior.

The occupational therapist worked with the teacher on introducing use of an incline board, a Movin' Sit™ cushion, a Thera-Band® under the desk, the fidget, and the sensory diet into the classroom. She explained his need for exercise breaks and coached the teacher to help him recognize the warning signs and to reward on-task behavior with the same frequency and attention that his out-of-seat and extraneous movements had previously warranted. He quickly improved, and the teacher found that she did not have to reinforce him as frequently for working quietly. She was able to fade the immediate gratification to a more intermittent reinforcement.

The Outcome

The teacher noted an immediate change in Adam's out-of-seat behaviors. Her ability to reward the in-seat behaviors resulted in less opportunity for attention from his peers and an increase in his self-esteem. The teacher felt empowered, understood his behaviors, and had concrete strategies to help him. Adam's skills improved over the next three months. He started to develop the internal postural control he needed to sit quietly in his chair. He also started to realize how vestibular and proprioceptive input helped him learn and process at school. He became aware of his state of arousal, need for constant stimulation, and of acceptable strategies to use in his seat. His occupational therapy treatment continued for the next year to further develop his fine and gross motor control, his skills and his ability to self-regulate. He went on to complete the year with a high B average and was promoted to the third grade.

The answer to the parents' original question "Is it behavior or is it sensory?" is that it was sensory. Adam's behavior was for productive sensory-obtaining reasons.

Case Study: Grace

12

Mary M. Murray, Ed.D.

Grace was born at thirty-two weeks' gestation. She was in the neonatal intensive care unit for six weeks to regulate her body temperature and heart rate. She also needed assistance to coordinate her suck, swallow, and breathing patterns. She was discharged home on an apnea monitor. She was evaluated for early intervention services at one month adjusted age, or three months chronological age. She qualified for services due to delays in communication skills (she was not making any sounds) and self-help skills (her feeding was labored and uncoordinated). An early-intervention specialist came to the home one day a week to work with Grace and her mother on communication and oral-motor skills. At 2.6 years of chronological age, Grace was discharged from early intervention and her parents were told that she "was caught up" and would do fine in preschool if she enrolled the next school year.

Grace has been enrolled in a private preschool three mornings a week since 3.6 years of age. There are fourteen children in the class, all three and four years old; one teacher; and a parent helper. The teacher has the room divided into centers. There is a carpeted quiet area with a bathtub filled with books in the middle of the carpet. There is also an area for manipulatives, a gross motor or play area, a sensory area with a variety of textures, a science area, an art area, and a carpeted semicircle used for "circle time." There is a bathroom in the classroom.

The first month seemed to go smoothly. The teacher told Grace's parents that she was doing fine in school and that she was a very active little girl. Then the preschool experience began to fall apart.

Grace generally walks into the classroom each morning and begins to cry while attempting to take off her coat. The parent helper assists her. She tries to hang her coat up on the hook underneath her cubby: It always falls down, and Grace cries and throws herself on the ground. The parent helper assists her hand-over-hand. The children are expected to find an activity and play until all of the other children have arrived. Grace walks aimlessly around the room kicking children's blocks and hitting anything she touches, including other children, until she is directed to an activity. Once the activity is demonstrated to Grace she will imitate the activity for up to five minutes at a time, as long as she can stand while completing the activity. While standing, Grace's feet move constantly and her body moves from side to side in a rhythmic motion. When Grace is "done" with one activity she will then wander around the room kicking and hitting until she is directed to another activity.

The teacher has noticed that Grace will fall on the floor screaming when she is in the art area if she did not put on a smock and the water or paint gets on her clothing. She screams while attempting to disrobe. Once she is assisted in changing the soiled clothing, she calms. Grace will not participate in any art activity that involves finger paint, pudding, shaving cream, or other similar textures. She will not self-select the texture tables unless water is the media. If any of these media (other than water) touch her hands, she will scream and throw herself on the floor until someone assists her up and helps her wash her hands.

Grace will interact with other children by imitating what they are doing. She has been heard to say about a hundred different words. She says most of her words during music activities. During circle time, which Grace enjoys, she will not sit, but will stand and perform most of the motions to many of the songs and will finger play. She screams when she is asked to sit down like the other children. The parent helper removes Grace from the situation when she screams. Grace enjoys washing her hands, swinging, rocking on the horse, and jumping on the trampoline. Grace will seek out the Sit and Spin® and initiate spinning. The teacher has noticed that she is able to stay with an activity for as long as ten minutes after she has been on the Sit and Spin® and when she comes in from recess. She does not like to transition from any of these activities.

The teacher has requested a meeting with the parents and the preschool director. She has mentioned to the parents that Grace is not appropriate for her preschool because she cannot follow the daily routine and is disruptive in the classroom. The teacher states that in order for Grace to stay in preschool, she must stop disrupting others with her hitting, kicking, screaming, and falling to the floor. The parents ask the teacher, "Is it sensory or is it behavior?"

In order to better assess each of her behaviors, we have looked at each separately and evaluated the behaviors in the figures at the end of this chapter. A blank Analyzing Behavior Worksheet is located in appendix D.

Behavior 1

Step 1. Identify and define the behavior:

- *Definition of behavior:* Kicks or hits others.

- *Priority for change?* Harmful to self and others. High priority for change.

Step 2. Look at the antecedent:

- *When does the behavior occur?*

  The behavior occurs only during unstructured, free time.

- *In what environments does the behavior occur?*

  Size of room does not appear to make a difference.

  Adult-to-child ratio does not appear to make a difference.

  Time of day is not a factor.

  Transitions do not seem to trigger the behavior.

- *Are there any recent special events?* None.

- *What are the warning signs that the behavior is about to occur?*

  Restlessness; child wandering around the room.

Antecedent is unstructured, free time.

Step 3. What is the primary cause of the behavior?

- *Is Grace trying to obtain something?* No.

- *Is Grace trying to avoid something?*

   In a manner of speaking, she avoids selecting and engaging in an activity when left to her own methods.

   One could say this is an example of task avoidance, but why? Certainly not for sensory reasons. In doing a task analysis, we find that when we demonstrate an activity to her, she is able to engage and imitate for five minutes or more.

   However, a skills analysis reveals that she lacks the ability to select an activity from the environment and initiate appropriate play. Grace has no idea of what to do or how to do it. She is avoiding tasks because they have no meaning to her. She has no idea what to do with the tasks. These skills fall under the umbrella of motor planning difficulties and must be addressed through a therapy intervention program. She is lost in her ability to find something to play with and to begin. She requires assistance to do this.

- *Is her method socially acceptable?*

   Certainly not. We must find a method for her to make a selection and engage in an activity before being allowed to wander around the room kicking or hitting others.

- *Is her method of communication acceptable?* No.
   - She lacks the ability to request help, or to make a selection.
   - We must identify a method by which she can choose an activity and ask for help.
   - We must teach her to use the communication systems.
   - We must reward any attempts she makes.

- *Are the behaviors linked?*

   Yes, they seem to occur together and appear to be caused by the same motor planning problems.

Step 4. What is the consequence to the behavior?

- *What happened after the behavior?*

   Immediately upon hitting or kicking another child, Grace receives attention from an adult and assistance in engaging and directing herself in a task.

- *What promotes the behavior?*

   The success she derives in getting the help she needs is what promotes the behavior, the primary reinforcer. It works for her.

   The secondary reinforcer to the behaviors is the attention she receives once she hits or kicks someone.

Step 5. What is the action plan?

- We want to stop the behavior by teaching her to ask for help in a socially acceptable method.

- We may offer her either an object reference or picture schedule of activities to do when she arrives in the morning or during "free time."

- We want to modify the task by making selections and engaging her in the selections before the behaviors erupt.

- A sensory diet is not needed to address these behaviors.

- Secondary reinforcers that might be used include praise and attention from an adult. A primary reinforcer, such as candy or the Sit and Spin®, should be used initially when teaching a new skill such as communication or a replacement behavior for wandering aimlessly. To establish the new behaviors, every time she engages in a task or asks for help, she must be reinforced.

- What consequences will there be? Our goal will be to attend to and reward on-task behaviors and communication; therefore, to extinguish the kicking and hitting, we must ignore it. We must block or redirect her when she attempts to hit or kick someone while not giving direct eye contact or verbal admonishments.

- Behavioral strategies will include predicting the behavior; stopping or blocking the behavior before it occurs or at its onset, and engaging her in an acceptable activity. Reward with attention and praise.

Behavior 2

Step 1. Identify and define the behavior:

- *Definition of behavior*: Throws self to floor.

- *Priority for change?* Harmful to self and others and is disruptive. High priority for change.

Step 2. Look at the antecedent:

- *When does the behavior occur?*

  The behavior occurs during art when she does not put on a smock and the water or paint gets on her clothing (undesirable sensory input) and when her coat falls to the ground (things do not go her way).

- *In what environments does the behavior occur?*

  Size of room does not appear to make a difference.

  Adult-to-child ratio does not appear to make a difference.

  Time of day is not a factor.

  Transitions do not seem to trigger the behavior.

- *Are there any recent special events?* None.

- *What are the warning signs that the behavior is about to occur?*

  When things do not go "right" for Grace or she does not like the sensory activity, she gets upset and throws herself to the floor.

Antecedent is undesirable sensory input or when unexpected mishaps occur.

Step 3: What is the primary cause of the behavior?

- *Is Grace trying to obtain something?* No.

- *Is Grace trying to avoid something?* Yes, but it is not immediately clear what that something is.

  1. She appears to have a sensory component to her behavior because she will avoid touching any media in art other than water, a colorless, odorless substance. The most probable reason may be a tactile defensiveness (hypersensitivity to touch), but olfactory (smell) defensiveness cannot be ruled out at this time. We must prepare her nervous system to be better able to handle the sensory activities. This can be done by:

     - A sensory diet of calming vestibular and deep-touch or proprioceptive input interspersed throughout the day.

     - Preparation activities before art, which should include heavy work especially to the hands. If tolerated, deep massages and toweling to the hands and arms would be helpful.

  2. A task analysis of each of the activities shows that she:

     - Has to reach the coat hook successfully to hang her coat.

     - Is using paint in easy-to-tip containers.

  3. A skills analysis reveals that the tasks are too difficult for her skill level. She lacks the skill to successfully motor plan, or hold her coat and direct it over the coat hook. In art, a skill analysis reveals that she does not grade the pressure on the containers and therefore cannot prevent water and other media from spilling on her. We must alter the tasks to ensure that she can be successful. We must:

     - Alter how or where she places her coat or offer assistance.

     - Work with media that is less apt to drip on her.

       We may choose a thickened liquid.

       We may use a spillproof or weighted container.

       We may use hand-over-hand assistance to ensure that the media does not spill.

     - We also must make sure that she dons a work smock before attempting art. Using an old shirt that has paint smudges on it may mask new drips and avoid the behaviors.

- There is another component to this behavior because the behavior occurs when she is frustrated or unsuccessful. When her coat falls to the floor or when something spills on her she perceives failure and reacts by throwing herself to the floor. This is a learned behavior to express her frustration and displeasure. Some of her screaming behaviors are linked to throwing herself on the floor. Others are not.

- *Is her method socially acceptable?* No, it is not.

  - We must help her understand what she is feeling.

  - We must redirect her to try again and assist her in being successful.

  - Praise her for her efforts.

- *Is her method of communication acceptable?* No.
  - Ensure that she has a way to ask for help.
  - We must allow her to express how she feels (i.e., "I'm mad").
- *Are the behaviors linked?*

  Yes. Throwing herself to the floor is often linked to crying and screaming behaviors.

Step 4: What is the consequence to the behavior?

- *What happened after the behavior?*

  When she throws herself to the floor she is immediately attended to, assisted up, and efforts are made to appease her. Her coat gets hung up for her, her clothing gets changed, and she is removed from art.

- *What promotes the behavior?*

  The immediate termination of the task is the primary reinforcer that promotes the behavior.

- The one-on-one attention she derives is the secondary reinforcer to the behavior.

Step 5: What is the action plan?

- We want to stop the behavior from being used.
- There are some environmental changes that can be made in art to make the behavior less apt to happen. See recommendations above.
- Teach communication: "I'm mad," "Help, please." Teach Grace to recognize what she is feeling.
- Modify the task and assist while remediating the skills needed for each task.
- Intervene before she hangs her coat; make her don a work smock before art; and assist with handling art materials.
- Establish a sensory diet to ward off defensiveness.
  - Swinging, the rocking horse, the Sit and Spin®, and jumping on the trampoline are alerting and organizing to her. Intersperse them throughout the day when organization and arousal is needed.
  - Heavy work and resistive tasks are calming. Intersperse when she needs to calm down and relax.
  - Before art, do heavy work activities. If tolerated, do deep-touch input to the arms and hands, such as deep massages, toweling, or brushing to the hands.
- Reinforce appropriate behavior using secondary reinforcers of praise and attention, or primary reinforcers which may include the Sit and Spin®.
- The consequences of the behavior must be that the tasks are not terminated. We must ignore her when she throws herself on the floor, then redirect her back to the task, and assist her in being successful.

Behavior 3

Step 1. Identify and define the behavior :

- *Definition of behavior:* Screaming and crying behavior.

- *Priority for change?* Disruptive; interferes with learning. Also not socially acceptable.

Step 2. Look at the antecedent:

- *When does the behavior occur?*

  Grace cries and screams at various times of the day. She cries when asked to take off her coat; she screams when her coat falls to the floor after she attempts to hang it up; and she screams when something spills on her in art or when she is asked to sit at circle time.

  The screaming that occurs when her coat falls and in art when something spills on her are linked to throwing herself on the floor and will be dealt with as explained in behavior number two.

- *In what environments does the behavior occur?*

  Size of room does not appear to make a difference.

  Adult to child ratio does not appear to make a difference.

  Circle time is the time when her screaming can be predicted. Grace likes standing and moving during circle time and always screams when asked to sit like the other children.

  Transitions do not seem to trigger the behavior.

- *Are there any recent special events?* None.

- *What are the warning signs that the behavior is about to occur?*

  Grace does not want to sit at circle time.

Antecedent is circle time.

Step 3. What is the primary cause of the behavior?

- *Is Grace trying to obtain something?*

  Yes, she wants to obtain movement during circle time. She enjoys performing the movement to the songs.

- *Is her method socially acceptable?* No.

  1. We must allow her movement during circle time. Perhaps she can sit on a rocking chair or inflatable cushion or be allowed to stand during the songs and participate in the movement that goes along with the songs.

  2. We may choose to have her sit in between songs and offer reinforcers when successful.

  Gradually increase her in-seat time between reinforcers.

- *Is her method of communication acceptable?* No.

  1. Ensure that she has a way to ask for permission to stand. When she uses communication, rather than screaming, allow her to stand.

  2. Ensure that she has a way to ask for certain songs.

Step 4. What is the consequence to the behavior?

- *What happened after the behavior?*

  When Grace screams at circle time, she is immediately removed from the group situation and the task is terminated.

- *What promotes the behavior?*

  Grace is demanding movement during circle time and screams when not allowed to have it. Note that she must also stand and move during activities once engaged. There are several possibilities to be considered here:

  1. Grace has made a rule that you stand and move to music. If that is the case, we must begin to alter the rule and expect her to cry or scream initially. We know Grace likes circle time. She may be allowed to stay for circle time if she sits either in between songs or on a moveable surface during circle time.

  2. The fact that Grace must stand to imitate activities and moves her feet constantly while sustaining an activity is a clue that she may lack the slow sustained postural control to remain seated while engaging her hands in an activity. She will need exercises and activities to strengthen her trunk and increase her muscle tone.

  3. Grace's need for movement also suggests that she may require movement (vestibular input) to regulate or modulate her level of arousal for the task.

  4. Regardless of the underlying cause, the fact that movement is productive for her and allows her to function is what promotes the behavior.

Step 5. What is the action plan?

- We must stop the behavior.

- Environmental changes may include the use of a rocking chair or cushion during circle time.

- Communication strategies may include verbal or pictorial strategies.

- Modifications to circle time may include having Grace sit between songs and then increasing in-seat time. They may also include use of a Movin' Sit™ or Sit and Fit cushion or some other inflatable cushion when she is attempting to imitate others in activities.

- A sensory diet is required that will include regular exercise or movement periods to modulate her level of arousal and improve postural mechanisms and control.

  - The vestibular input of the sit and spin and rocking horse will increase her arousal and muscle tone.

  - The trampoline (vestibular and proprioceptive input) often has an arousing and calming effect.

  - Heavy work and resistive activities will calm, organize, and strengthen her.

- Reinforcers may be the movement or exercise periods themselves as well as praise and attention for on-task behavior. Bouncing her on a ball or inflatable cushion while seated when she attempts an activity may be used as a reinforcer.

- Consequences may include:

    1. Delaying the next song in circle time until she sits momentarily.

    2. Consequences for screaming when asked to sit to perform an activity must be that she be redirected and assisted to complete minimal requirements in the activity before being allowed out of her seat and termination of the task.

- Behavioral strategies that may be used might include ignoring (not acknowledging the screams) while directing her to on-task behavior and rewarding immediately. Positive behavioral momentum would also be effective to get in-seat behavior in order to reward her.

- Sensory strategies might include allowing movement at regular intervals and as a reward to aid in her postural control and organization. This will aid in eliminating her need to scream and cry.

Analyzing Behavior Worksheet

Child's name _Grace_

Behavior _(Example 1) Kicking or hitting_

Date _____

Define the behavior: _Kicks or hits others_

Are Behaviors Linked? (Yes/No)

☐ Y ☒ N Stem from the same cause?

☐ Y ☒ N Occur in a predictable pattern?

Group behaviors with the same cause together.

Analyze behaviors with the same underlying cause as one behavior (a single entity).

Priority for change:

☒ Harmful to self or others

☐ Destructive

☐ Disruptive/Interferes with learning

☐ Not acceptable (socially)

Action Plan

☒ Stop

☐ Alter

☐ Limit or modify the behavior

☐ Ignore

☐ Treat the underlying problem

Antecedent: Is it a problem? (Yes/No)

☐ Y ☒ N Size of room

☒ Y ☐ N Structured/unstructured task

☐ Y ☒ N Adult-child ratio?

☐ Y ☒ N Environmental factors: Noise/clutter/other

☐ Y ☒ N Time of day:

☒ Y ☐ N Morning/evening/transitions?

☒ Y ☐ N During certain activities?

Characteristics of activity:

unstructured tasks

What activity or event preceded the behavior?

_N/A_

Action Plan

Environmental changes needed:

Picture Schedule or other method of directing child.

Recent special events

☐ Illness

☐ Lack of sleep

☐ Family dispute

☐ Other:

☒ None

Action Plan

Is a referral to a professional indicated?

Warning signs

☒ Restlessness

☐ Eye aversion

☐ Distractibility

☐ Pause

☐ Raises voice

☐ Self-stimulation or repetitive pattern: Describe behavior

☐ Other: _Unstructured time_

Action Plan

Can you intervene at this point to ward off the behavior? _Yes._
Give structured task or have an adult with the child.

Figure 12.1   Analyzing behavior worksheet: kicking behavior

Analyzing Behavior Worksheet (continued)

Child's name _Grace_

Date _____

Behavior (_Example 1) Kicking or hitting_

Define the behavior: _Kicks or hits others_

Primary cause: Obtain _N/A_

- ☐ Attention
- ☐ Object
- ☐ Need
- ☐ Want
- ☐ Activity
- ☐ Sensory
  - ☐ productive
  - ☐ nonproductive

Does it work for the child?

Is the child successful in obtaining what he wants/needs?

Action Plan _N/A_

Identify a method to get what the child wants as part of his normal schedule, as a reward, etc.

Primary Cause: Avoid

- ☐ Attention
  - ☐ positive
  - ☐ negative
- ☐ People
- ☐ Situations
- ☐ Transitions
- ☒ Task, object or activity
  Avoids selecting and engaging in an activity

Action Plan

Perform task analysis

- ☒ Task too difficult?
- ☐ Task not stimulating?
- ☐ Not challenging?
- ☐ Task boring?
- ☐ Difficulty adjusting to transition?
- ☐ Task overwhelming?
- ☐ Dislikes task?
- ☐ Lacks self-confidence?
- ☐ Fears task?
- ☐ Avoids sensory aspect?
- ☒ Task has no meaning?

Perform skills analysis

Does child have the necessary skills to do the task? _No_

If not, how will you remediate? _physical resistance_
Analyze emotional response

If child has necessary skills, give emotional support and physical assistance.

Primary Cause: Avoiding Sensory _N/A_
(Internal Systemic)

What type of sensory input?

- ☐ Vestibular
- ☐ Auditory
- ☐ Visual
- ☐ Smell
- ☐ Tactile

Is it systemic/visceral due to:

- ☐ Pain or discomfort?
- ☐ Hunger?
- ☐ Illness or impending illness?
- ☐ Hot, tired, sweaty?
- ☐ Other: _____

Is he avoiding something sensory from the environment? Identify the cause:

Action Plan _N/A_

1. Identify if sensory and how you will remediate.

2. If based upon a need, can you rectify it?

Social and Communication—Aspects of Behavior

- ☐ Y ☒ N **Is it socially acceptable?**
  If not, identify other methods.
- ☐ Y ☒ N **Is method of communication acceptable?**
  If not, must address communication strategies.

Primary Causes: Action Plan

- ☒ Socially Acceptable Behaviors: Teach
- ☒ Communication Strategies: Identify and teach
- ☒ Task: Alter, modify, or assist
- ☒ Skills: Teach or develop skills
- ☐ Sensory Options:
  - ☐ Enhance the sensory component
  - ☐ Decrease sensory component
  - ☐ Provide sensory diets
  - ☐ Provide scheduled sensory activities
- ☐ Environmental Modifications:

Figure 12.1   Analyzing behavior worksheet: kicking behavior (continued)

Analyzing Behavior Worksheet (continued)

Behavior (_Example 1) Kicking or hitting_

Define the behavior: _Kicks or hits others_

Consequence to Behavior:

What predicts the behavior?
Unstructured time

What promotes the behavior?
attention and assistance

What happened after the behavior?
She is given attention and direction

What are consequences to behavior?
attention and assistance

What is primary cause?
Child may not have an idea of what to do (motor planning problems)

What is primary reinforcer?
success in getting help

What are secondary reinforcers?
attention

Action Plan

What behavior do you want to occur? _Child should ask for help with activity. She should ask for help with activity selection & to independently engage in activities._

Stop/Alter/Limit/Modify the Behavior/Do nothing or treat the underlying cause.
Modify the behavior.
Teach to ask for help.

Environmental changes needed?
Picture schedule.

What communication strategies are needed?
Picture schedule.

What modifications to task and skills will you make?
1) Structure tasks
2) Make task easier for her to engage in.

When will you intervene?
Before any free time.

Is a sensory diet needed?
Not for this behavior.

What reinforcers will you use? _1) Attention and praise_
2) Primary reinforcer for new behavior (candy, Sit and Spin)

What consequences will there be?
Ignore the behavior & redirect to another activity.

What behavioral strategies will you use?
Stop the behavior: predict it and encourage the child before behavior occurs

Do you need to refer the child for other services? _Yes_
OT or PT for sensory integration therapy or other services? (OT or PT to improve her motor planning)

Figure 12.1   Analyzing behavior worksheet: kicking behavior (continued)

Analyzing Behavior Worksheet

Child's name __Grace__

Behavior __(Example 2) Throwing self to Floor__   Date _____

Define the behavior: _Throws self to floor_
a) when her coat drops
b) in art when something gets on her clothing
c) when things don't go right—something unexpected occurs

Are Behaviors Linked? (Yes/No)

☐ Y ☒ N Stem from the same cause?

☐ Y ☒ N Occur in a predictable pattern?

Group behaviors with the same cause together.

Analyze behaviors with the same underlying cause as one behavior (a single entity).

Priority for change:

☐ Harmful to self or others

☒ Destructive

☐ Disruptive/Interferes with learning

☒ Not acceptable (socially)

Action Plan

☒ Stop

☐ Alter

☐ Limit or modify the behavior

☐ Ignore

☐ Treat the underlying problem

Antecedent: Is it a problem? (Yes/No)

☐ Y ☒ N Size of room

☐ Y ☒ N Structured/unstructured task

☐ Y ☒ N Adult-child ratio?

☐ Y ☒ N Environmental factors: Noise/clutter/other

☐ Y ☒ N Time of day:

☐ Y ☒ N Morning/evening/transitions?

☒ Y ☐ N During certain activities?

Characteristics of activity:
1) hanging her coat
2) paint gets on her clothing

What activity or event preceded the behavior?

Things don't go as expected or correctly.

Action Plan

Environmental changes needed: _No_

Recent special events

☐ Illness

☐ Lack of sleep

☐ Family dispute

☐ Other:

☒ None

Action Plan

Is a referral to a professional indicated?

Warning signs

☐ Restlessness

☐ Eye aversion

☐ Distractibility

☐ Pause

☐ Raises voice

☐ Self-stimulation or repetitive pattern: Describe behavior

☐ Other: _When she is unsuccessful or things don't go as expected_

Action Plan

Can you intervene at this point to ward off the behavior? _Yes._
Offer assistance with tasks.

Figure 12.2   Analyzing behavior worksheet: throwing self to floor

Analyzing Behavior Worksheet (continued)

Behavior _(Example 2) Throwing self to Floor_

Define the behavior: Throws self to floor
a) when her coat drops
b) in art when something gets on her clothing
c) when things don't go right-something unexpected occurs

Primary cause: Obtain N/A	**Primary Cause: Avoid**	**Primary Cause: Avoiding Sensory** N/A (Internal Systemic)	**Social and Communication—Aspects of Behavior**
☐ Attention	☐ Attention	What type of sensory input?	☐ Y ☒ N **Is it socially acceptable?**
☐ Object	☐ positive	☐ Vestibular	If not, identify other methods.
☐ Need	☐ negative	☐ Auditory	
☐ Want	☐ People	☐ Visual	☐ Y ☒ N **Is method of communication acceptable?**
☐ Activity	☐ Situations	☒ Smell	
☐ Sensory	☐ Transitions	☒ Tactile	If not, must address communication strategies.
☐ productive	☒ Task, object or activity	Is it systemic/visceral due to:	
☐ nonproductive		☐ Pain or discomfort?	

Does it work for the child?

Action Plan

Perform task analysis

☒ Task too difficult?
☐ Task not stimulating?
☐ Not challenging?
☐ Task boring?
☐ Difficulty adjusting to transition?
☐ Task overwhelming?
☐ Dislikes task?
☐ Lacks self-confidence?
☐ Fears task?
☒ Avoids sensory aspect? _Art_
☐ Task has no meaning? _media?_

Perform skills analysis

Does child have the necessary skills to do the task? _No_

If not, how will you remediate?
teach skills and refer to OT
Analyze emotional response

If child has necessary skills, give emotional support and physical assistance. _Yes_

Is the child successful in obtaining what he wants/needs?

Action Plan   N/A

Identify a method to get what the child wants as part of his normal schedule, as a reward, etc.

(Primary Cause: Avoiding Sensory column, continued)
☐ Hunger?
☐ Illness or impending illness?
☐ Hot, tired, sweaty?
☐ Other: _____

Is he avoiding something sensory from the environment? Identify the cause:

Action Plan

1. Identify if sensory and how you will remediate. _Sensory Diet to avoid defensiveness, and refer to a sensory integration trained therapist to address the underlying sensory and motor planning issues._

2. If based upon a need, can you rectify it?

Primary Causes: Action Plan

☒ Socially Acceptable Behaviors: Teach
☒ Communication Strategies: Identify and teach
☒ Task: Alter, (modify) or (assist)
☒ Skills: Teach or develop skills
☒ Sensory Options:
  ☐ Enhance the sensory component
  ☒ Decrease sensory component
  ☒ Provide sensory diets
  ☐ Provide scheduled sensory activities
☐ Environmental Modifications:

Figure 12.2   Analyzing behavior worksheet: throwing self to floor (continued)

Child's name ___Grace___   Date ___

Analyzing Behavior Worksheet (continued)

Behavior ___(Example 2) Throwing self to Floor___

Define the behavior: *Throws self to floor*
a) *when her coat drops*
b) *in art when something gets on her clothing*
c) *when things don't go right—something unexpected occurs*

Consequence to Behavior:	**Action Plan**
What predicts the behavior? *FRUSTRATION*	What behavior do you want to occur? *child will communicate her frustration; ask for help; work in a variety of art media with assistance*
	(Stop)/Alter/Limit/Modify the Behavior/Do nothing or treat the underlying cause.
What promotes the behavior?	
one-to-one attention, task assistance, or task termination	Environmental changes needed? *Modify media and containers used in art.*
What happened after the behavior?	What communication strategies are needed? *devise a system; teach and reinforce its use.*
one-to-one attention, task assistance, or task avoidance	What modifications to task and skills will you make? *assist for modify tasks*
What are consequences to behavior?	When will you intervene? 1) *Before she hangs her coat;*
attention, assistance, task avoidance	2) *Before art to put on smock and to assist in handling the media.*
What is primary cause? *Lacks skills. She may lack skills needed for some tasks, but may have learned an emotional response to certain more difficult tasks & need emotional support.*	Is a sensory diet needed? *yes*
What is primary reinforcer?	What reinforcers will you use? *Sit and Spin*
task avoidance	What consequences will there be? *Ignore the behaviors; redirect to task*
assistance gained attention	What behavioral strategies will you use? 1) *Reinforce appropriate behaviors, 2)Ignore the throwing self to floor, and 3) Redirect to task.*
What are secondary reinforcers?	Do you need to refer the child for other services?
attention	OT or PT for sensory integration therapy or other services? *Yes*

Figure 12.2   Analyzing behavior worksheet: throwing self to floor (continued)

Analyzing Behavior Worksheet

Child's name ___Grace___   Date _____

Behavior ___Example 3 Screaming & crying___

Define the behavior: Screaming and crying:
a) when asked to sit at circle time or at other seated tasks e.g., fine motor
b) when asked to take coat off & it falls to floor. This behavior is linked to throwing herself to floor & is dealt with under Ex. 2.

Are Behaviors Linked? (Yes/No)

☒Y ☐N Stem from the same cause? *Hanging coat up*

☒Y ☐N Occur in a predictable pattern?

Group behaviors with the same cause together. *Screaming or crying when asked to take coat off and it falls to floor, is linked to throwing self on floor. It is dealt with in example 2.*

Analyze behaviors with the same underlying cause as one behavior (a single entity).

Priority for change:

☐ Harmful to self or others

☐ Destructive

☒ Disruptive/Interferes with learning

☒ Not acceptable (socially)

Action Plan

☒ Stop

☐ Alter

☐ Limit or modify the behavior

☐ Ignore

☐ Treat the underlying problem

Antecedent: Is it a problem? (Yes/No)

☐Y ☒N Size of room

☐Y ☒N Structured/unstructured task

☐Y ☒N Adult-child ratio?

☐Y ☒N Environmental factors: Noise/clutter/other

☐Y ☒N Time of day:

☒Y ☐N Morning/evening/transitions? *circle time*

☒Y ☐N During certain activities?
Characteristics of activity: *seated activities*

What activity or event preceded the behavior? *N/A*

Action Plan

Environmental changes needed:
Add an inflatable cushion or rocking chair to circle time. Use inflatable cushion for fine motor & other seated activities.

Action Plan

Is a referral to a professional indicated?
Child is a candidate for OT/PT evaluation

Warning signs

☐ Restlessness

☐ Eye aversion

☐ Distractibility

☐ Pause

☒ Raises voice

☐ Self-stimulation or repetitive pattern: Describe behavior

☐ Other:

Action Plan

Can you intervene at this point to ward off the behavior? *Yes*

Figure 12.3   Analyzing behavior worksheet: screaming and crying

Analyzing Behavior Worksheet (continued)

Child's name _Grace_

Date _____

Behavior _Example 3 Screaming & crying_

Define the behavior: _Screaming & crying when asked to sit at circle time or other seated tasks e.g., fine motor._

Primary cause: Obtain	**Primary Cause: Avoid** _N/A_	**Primary Cause: Avoiding Sensory** _N/A_ (Internal Systemic)	**Social and Communication—Aspects of Behavior**
☐ Attention	☐ Attention	What type of sensory input?	☐ Y ☒ N **Is it socially acceptable?**
☐ Object	☐ positive	☐ Vestibular	If not, identify other methods.
☐ Need	☐ negative	☐ Auditory	
☐ Want	☐ People	☐ Visual	☐ Y ☒ N **Is method of communication acceptable?**
☐ Activity	☐ Situations	☐ Smell	
☒ Sensory _wants to obtain_	☐ Transitions	☐ Tactile	If not, must address communication strategies.
☒ productive _movement_	☐ Task, object or activity	Is it systemic/visceral due to:	
☐ nonproductive		☐ Pain or discomfort?	
Does it work for the child? _Yes, it increases arousal and muscle tone so that she is better able to attend and perform._	**Action Plan** _N/A_	☐ Hunger?	
	Perform task analysis	☐ Illness or impending illness?	
	☐ Task too difficult?	☐ Hot, tired, sweaty?	**Primary Causes: Action Plan**
	☐ Task not stimulating?	☐ Other: _____	☒ Socially Acceptable Behaviors: Teach and teach
	☐ Not challenging?	Is he avoiding something sensory from the environment? Identify the cause: _No_	☒ Communication Strategies: Identify and teach
Is the child successful in obtaining what he wants/needs?	☐ Task boring?		☐ Task: Alter, modify, or assist
	☐ Difficulty adjusting to transition?		☐ Skills: Teach or develop skills
Yes	☐ Task overwhelming?	**Action Plan** _N/A_	☐ Sensory Options:
	☐ Dislikes task?	1. Identify if sensory and how you will remediate.	☒ Enhance the sensory component
	☐ Lacks self-confidence?		☐ Decrease sensory component
	☐ Fears task?		☐ Provide sensory diets
	☐ Avoids sensory aspect?		☐ Provide scheduled sensory activities
	☐ Task has no meaning?		☒ Environmental Modifications:
Action Plan	**Perform skills analysis**	2. If based upon a need, can you rectify it?	_Add a cushion or rocking chair for seated tasks._
Identify a method to get what the child wants as part of his normal schedule, as a reward, etc.	Does child have the necessary skills to do the task?		
Build movement into activities	If not, how will you remediate?		
	Analyze emotional response		
	If child has necessary skills, give emotional support and physical assistance.		

Figure 12.3 Analyzing behavior worksheet: screaming and crying (continued)

Analyzing Behavior Worksheet (continued)

Define the behavior: *Screaming & crying when asked to sit at circle time or other seated tasks e.g., fine motor.*

Consequence to Behavior:	Action Plan
What predicts the behavior?	**What behavior do you want to occur?** *Grace will sit during*
circle time & other seated tasks	*circle time, ask to stand to dance or perform during some songs.*
	Stop/Alter/Limit/Modify the Behavior/Do nothing or treat the underlying cause.
What promotes the behavior?	*STOP/Avoid the need for screaming & crying.*
Movement is productive for Grace.	**Environmental changes needed?** *Provide movement for seated activities e.g., rocking chair or inflatable cushion.*
What happened after the behavior?	
Task terminated & avoided.	**What communication strategies are needed?**
	verbal & pictorial
What are consequences to behavior?	**What modifications to task and skills will you make?**
Task avoidance	*1) Have her sit between songs at circle time*
movement allowed.	*2) Use inflatable cushion for seated tasks.*
	When will you intervene?
What is primary cause?	*Before circle time & during other seated tasks. Encourage on-task behaviors.*
Grace requires movement in order to attend to & perform a seated task	**Is a sensory diet needed?**
	yes
What is primary reinforcer?	**What reinforcers will you use?**
Productive sensory–she gets to move out of her seat.	*(vestibular) movement and praise*
	What consequences will there be?
What are secondary reinforcers?	*Grace will return to task.*
Task termination/avoidance & perhaps attention.	**What behavioral strategies will you use?** *Use positive behavioral momentum to get seated; do not acknowledge crying or screaming. Assist to redirect in-seat activity; reward on-task behaviors immediately. Provide opportunities for sensory diet.*
	Do you need to refer the child for other services?
	OT or PT for sensory integration therapy or other services?
	Yes

Figure 12.3   Analyzing behavior worksheet: screaming and crying (continued)

Appendix A

Characteristics of Underresponsiveness to Tactile and Proprioceptive Input: Tactile Discrimination Difficulties

Tactile discrimination difficulties are characterized by an underresponsiveness to touch and proprioceptive input. The characteristics children may display will reflect their differences and personalities as well as the degree of integration within their nervous systems.

General Characteristics

Enjoys touch pressure (e.g., massage, being squeezed or held tight).

May not register or respond to hugging, cuddling, or tickling.

Does not notice food on face, runny nose, or messy hands.

Does not notice when pants are soiled, diapers are wet, or clothing has become undone or fallen off.

Is a messy dresser (e.g., shirt is seldom tucked in, shoes are untied, pants are twisted).

Needs to touch and feel everything; seeing it is not enough. Must run hands along the walls and over furniture, handle toys, test items, and so on.

Often bumps into and touches others. Has trouble keeping hands to self.

Shows little or no reaction to pain from scrapes, bruises, cuts, or injections.

Plays roughly with toys, objects, other children, adults, and animals.

Does not realize the degree of force exerted; may hurt others or break toys.

Does not understand the pain others can feel; may have no remorse for hurting others.

Likes to scratch or rub surfaces; may scratch or rub skin excessively; may bite self.

Dislikes the dark; needs to see surroundings.

May display motor planning difficulties (see chapter 2, Sensory Integration and Sensory Processing Disorders).

Total Body and Body Awareness Characteristics

Is unable to identify without looking where touched on the body.

Is not bothered by falls.

Enjoys crashing into other people, objects, mats, balls; likes to fall or throw self on or off equipment.

Enjoys intense sensory experiences, such as movements that provide strong sensory feedback: jumping from high places, vibration, crashing into things with great force.

(continued)

Characteristics of Underresponsiveness to Tactile and Proprioceptive Input: Tactile Discrimination Difficulties (*Continued*)

Is a safety risk; is unaware of physical danger to self.

Does not know where body parts are and how they relate to one another.

Does not appear to know that legs are connected to body.

    Does not use legs to stabilize self in a chair; frequently falls out of the chair.

    Legs appear awkward and uncoordinated when running.

Is not able to imitate new movements or learn through imitation.

Is awkward in attempts to get dressed.

    Has trouble orienting arms to go into a shirt, figuring out how to get feet into socks and shoes, and/or orienting pants and getting legs into them.

Is constantly in motion.

    Appears to excel in fast movements, but arms and legs lack coordination and midrange control.

    Uses only end ranges with poor grading of arm and leg movements.

    Does not have the slow, sustained postural control needed for slow movements.

    Runs from place to place, thing to thing; is unable to stay on task.

Is constantly climbing to high places; or does not have the motor control to climb or jump.

Has low muscle tone.

    Muscles seem mushy and inactive; may hyperextend midjoints and/or display a lordotic posture (rounding forward of shoulders with hyperextension of the lumbar spine and hyper-extension of the knees).

    Moving and playing require effort.

    Tires quickly with minimal exertion.

    Prefers sedentary activities, such as reading or watching videos or TV.

Fine-Motor Characteristics

Hands appear disconnected from the body: hands seem like unfamiliar appendages.

Hand movements are uncoordinated.

Lacks isolated finger control, in-hand manipulation skills, ability to oppose the thumb to each consecutive finger.

    Fingers move as a unit, as if child were wearing mittens.

    Cannot imitate finger movements; has difficulty showing thumbs-up, the peace sign, or number of years old on fingers.

    Has difficulty controlling the fingers for precise tasks.

Must visually monitor hand movements.

Drops things, but fails to realize when things are dropped.

(continued)

Characteristics of Underresponsiveness to Tactile and Proprioceptive Input: Tactile Discrimination Difficulties (*Continued*)

Has trouble identifying and understanding the physical properties of objects (e.g., textures, shapes, size, density, weight).

Is unable to identify familiar objects by touch alone.

    Must use vision when reaching into a desk, under a table, or in a box for an object.

    Cannot identify items in own pocket or get them out.

Uses mouth as a third hand to stabilize objects or hold them in order to help the hands.

Uses mouth to provide more sensory information about objects.

After age two, mouths objects to learn about the qualities of the object.

Has difficulty holding and using tools (e.g., crayons, pencils, scissors, spoons, forks).

Has learned to use the hands, but does so in strange ways; puts on socks, shoes, and/or gloves in unusual ways.

Oral-Motor Behaviors

Barely moves lips, cheeks, or tongue.

Cannot imitate tongue movements or facial expressions.

Facial expression appears flat; does not move cheeks or facial muscles to express emotions or during conversation.

Has difficulty sucking through a straw, blowing a whistle, and/or blowing kisses.

Bites the cup when trying to drink from it; bites the straw or whistle when blowing.

Does not move tongue much when talking or eating.

Drools.

Loses liquid when drinking from a cup.

Is a messy eater; appears unaware when face is messy or covered with crumbs of food, or liquid is dripping from mouth.

Stuffs the mouth with food when eating; does not appear to know there is food in the mouth unless it is packed.

Refuses to eat anything but familiar and comfortable foods or snacks.

Has definite food and drink preferences.

Must visually inspect any new foods or snacks; reacts to foods based on appearance, not on taste.

Cannot physically handle foods of varying textures or qualities; eats only familiar foods that are exactly the same size, texture, and quality.

Mouths everything (e.g., toys and objects, clothing, washcloths, towels).

Vocalizations lack variety.

Has articulation difficulties.

Intervention for Tactile Discrimination Disorders

- Use sensory stimulation to awaken the system: lotion massages, toweling extremities, brushing.

- Use activities that require tactile exploration both with and without vision.

- Move from tactile stimulation to tactile discrimination by encouraging the child to identify the tactile quality of objects without vision.

For the hands

- Find objects, without using vision, in rice, therapy putty, macaroni, beans, shaving cream.

- Provide resistance to hand and finger movements: use resistive clothespins, incline boards when writing, put sandpaper under the writing surface, therapy putty, and so on.

For the mouth

- Start with activities to awaken the mouth: use a Nuk® brush to stimulate the gums, tongue, and inside of the cheeks.

- Use resistive whistles to activate the muscles of the lips and cheek.

- Using the child's favorite foods with a variety of textures, place a small amount of food in the child's mouth and have him identify the food by taste and texture.

- Place three different types of pretzels in front of the child. Without allowing the child to see, place one of them in his mouth and have the child identify which one it is. Choose different types of foods.

For the feet

- Start with activities to stimulate the feet, such as lotion massages, toweling, or playing in textured objects.

- Use the toes to find objects hidden in sand, rice, or beans, then place them in a bucket.

- Walk on foam blocks, mats, or inflatable surfaces.

For the body

- Do resistive gross-motor activities for the total body. Resistance may be added through weights, resistive equipment, or using body weight against gravity.

- Starting with total body activities, work toward more skilled and precise movements.

- Encourage extracurricular activities that are resistive and enhance body scheme, such as bike riding, swimming, horseback riding, roller-blading/skating, karate, gymnastics, and ballet.

Appendix B

Intervention for Tactile Defensiveness

Limit the amount of tactile inputs through limited changes in hand placements and limited use of light touch. Let the child guide the type and amount of touch provided. Most children prefer firm touch rather than light touch.

Desensitize the tactile system

Utilize deep-touch pressure and proprioceptive inputs to calm the system.

Engage the child in heavy work to calm down the system.

- Weight-bearing exercises: arm pushups, handstands
- Isometric exercises
- Extracurricular activities: bike riding, skating, swimming, karate, climbing activities on playgrounds
- Household chores that are resistive

Assure that heavy work is interspersed throughout the day, as in a sensory diet.

Make environmental modifications

- Limit specific environmental stimulation that contributes to overarousal.
- Use inhibitory sensory inputs: darkened rooms, low volumes, quiet music.
- Decrease overstimulation.
- Provide structure.
- Use activities that are rhythmic and organizing.

Teach calming techniques and self-regulation. Teach the child:

- To identify warning signs of escalating stress levels.
- What his or her sensory needs are and what environments are difficult for him or her.

(continued)

Intervention for Tactile Defensiveness (Continued)

- Coping strategies, including:

  - Communication strategies

  - Sensory strategies to alter arousal levels, such as therapeutic listening (music)

  - Cognitive strategies

- Make a list of calming and organizing strategies that work. Prompt the child to use them in environments where they are needed.

- Provide verbal cues for calming.

Work on specific skills that are creating a problem, such as eating; dressing; socializing; and/or fine-motor, oral-motor, postural, or gross-motor skills.

Work through difficult tasks as described on the next pages.

Tactile Defensiveness: Intervention Strategies for Common Problems

Tactile defensiveness is an aversive or negative behavioral response to certain tactile stimuli that others do not find to be noxious. It includes avoidance of touch, aversive response to non-noxious touch, and atypical emotional responses to touch.

Problem	Intervention
Child hates having hair combed, washed, or cut.	■ Sit child firmly in your lap. Squeeze child between your knees (deep pressure).
	■ Place your hands on the child's head and exert gentle but firm downward pressure (joint compression of the neck inhibits defensiveness). During joint compression, you must have correct alignment of the head and spine.
	■ Use firm strokes or pressure as you comb or wash child's hair.
	■ Count or have the child count as you comb, wash, rinse, or cut hair.
	■ Give definite time limits to the task: "Let's count to ten. Then we will stop cutting your hair." Provide inhibition techniques immediately after.
	■ Break the task into each substep. This is effective for activities such as hair cuts.
	▪ Eliminate any unnecessary steps or items.
	▪ Use inhibition techniques (described above) while emotionally coaching the child through each step and familiarizing him or her with each item.
	▪ Practice each step in isolation in a stress-free environment.
	▪ Gradually combine steps and perform the task in the natural environment.
Child hates baths or showers.	■ Before bath time, do resistive exercises or activities that provide deep proprioceptive input.
	■ Have the bathwater drawn before the child undresses. Make the transition from undressing to entering the tub as quickly and smoothly as possible.
	■ If the child dislikes having his or her face or body washed, encourage the child to do it by himself or herself. Self-imposed touch produces a less defensive reaction.
	■ Use a large sponge or loofa sponge. Rub firmly to decrease defensiveness.
	■ Use fragrance-free soap made for sensitive skin.
	■ If the child is showering, use a handheld shower nozzle. Let the child control the direction and force of the water.
	■ Use a large towel, and quickly and firmly wrap the child in it. Avoid exposure of the wet skin to the air as the light touch may trigger a defensive reaction.
	■ Provide deep-touch toweling to the extremities, hands, and feet to decrease defensiveness. If the child will tolerate it, provide a firm massage, using lotion to avoid skin irritation.

(continued)

Tactile Defensiveness: Intervention Strategies for Common Problems (*Continued*)

Problem	Intervention
Child acts out when standing in line or starts to push and shove other children.	■ Position child at the end of the line. Others bumping against him or her may be threatening or painful.
	■ Assign a special task. Have the child go ahead to make sure the area is ready or stay behind to make sure the lights are turned off.
Child withdraws or punches others who touch him or her lightly.	■ Teach others to touch the child firmly. Discuss that the child feels light touch as alerting and as if he or she were being hit.
	■ Approach child from within his or her visual field.
Child reacts negatively when touched from behind or when touched by others.	■ Tell the child when you are going to touch him or her. Always touch firmly. Assure the child you will touch firmly and that you will not move your hands.
Child reacts negatively and emotionally to light touch (exhibits anxiety, hostility, or aggression).	■ Teach friends and relatives to show affection firmly and directly.
Child may pull away when approached for a friendly pat or caress from a relative or friend.	■ Tell the child what you will do and how you will do it. ("I'm going to hug you real hard.") Respect the child's need for control.
Child may crave the deep-touch pressure of a hug but try to rub off the light touch of a kiss.	■ Make kisses on the cheek a form of deep-touch input. Hold the child firmly and give a deep, firm kiss.
Child may reject touch altogether from anyone but his or her mother or primary caregiver.	■ Choose to give firm hugs rather than kisses. Take turns hugging. Have the child hug first, then return the hug. Determine who gives the best hugs.
Child may control when and by whom he is touched.	■ Teach people to always approach the child from the front and always to make sure the child is able to anticipate the hug or expression of affection.
An infant may reject cuddling as a source of pleasure and calming.	■ Swaddle child firmly. Be sensitive to the child's need for minimal sensory stimulation. Avoid vigorous rocking and shaking if he or she is upset. Rock slowly in a linear direction (up and down, side-to-side, or front-to-back). Swaddle and hold child firmly. Talk quietly and softly.
Infant may prefer the father's firm touch over the mother's light touch.	
Child is picky or dislikes certain clothing.	
Seams on socks are bothersome.	■ Turn socks inside out so seam is on outside; use seamless socks.
New clothing is irritating.	■ Wash new clothing to take out the stiffness. Have child help select clothing.
Tags on clothing are irritating.	■ Remove tags until the child's nervous system can tolerate them.
Child will only wear certain clothes.	■ Avoid buying clothing that the child perceives as irritating. The head, neck, and abdominal area are very sensitive to touch.
	■ Use inhibition techniques: Joint compression, deep-touch, proprioceptive input.

(continued)

Tactile Defensiveness: Intervention Strategies for Common Problems (*Continued*)

Problem	Intervention

Child takes off clothes inappropriately.	■ When child removes clothes because they are overstimulating or arousing:
	
	   ■ Use inhibitory techniques. Have the child wear snug or tight-fitting clothes.
	
	■ When the child removes clothes because he or she likes the feeling of the air on the skin:
	
	   ■ Have the child wear loose-fitting clothes for added touch.

Child is a picky eater. Child prefers certain textures. Child refuses to eat foods with lumps. Child dislikes sticky foods.	■ Place the child on an oral-motor program. ■ Before mealtime, provide deep-touch, resistive oral-motor and total-body exercises to decrease touch defensiveness. ■ Do not introduce new foods or challenges at mealtime. Set aside a separate time for graded feeding programs to remediate the underlying problem. Try to make mealtime a relaxed, pleasurable experience.
Child uses only his or her fingertips to play with toys, or handle crayons and pencils.	■ Before activities, provide phasic deep pressure into the palms of the hands, such as firm clapping or a modified donkey game in which you hold the child on your lap, face down, and parallel to the floor. Quickly lower the child to the floor, thus activating protective reactions (the child catches himself or herself on hands). ■ Progress to sustained deep pressure into the palms through resistive or weight-bearing activities. ■ Before activities, provide deep touch to the palms of the hand. Use firm brushing with a surgical scrub brush, or a deep massage followed by firm toweling. ■ Grade activities from using fingertips to the whole hand. If the child will tolerate it, provide deep-touch input over the hand and writing tool.

Child avoids getting hands dirty or using messy materials.
 	
Child hurries to wash off even a speck of dirt.
 	
Child may verbally rationalize why hands can't get dirty ("My mother won't let me").
	■ Encourage less messy activities.
	
	■ Use tools to manipulate the supplies whenever possible (for example, a paintbrush rather than fingerpaint).
	
	■ Before messy tasks:
	
	   ■ Use phasic deep pressure into the palms (described above).
	
	   ■ Use inhibitory techniques (deep-touch and proprioceptive input) to the hands and total body.
	
	   ■ Use messy materials that provide resistance, such as putties or dough mixtures.
	
	   ■ Provide external resistance to the child's arm movements.

(continued)

Tactile Defensiveness: Intervention Strategies for Common Problems (*Continued*)

Problem	Intervention
Child may toe-walk to avoid contact with the ground.	■ Check for heel-cord shortening. Range must be increased in order to decrease walking on tiptoes. ■ Provide deep pressure into the bottom of the feet. Seat the child firmly in your lap facing a wall. Place the child's feet flat against the wall and put pressure directly through the knees into the feet. Have the child help push. ■ Progress to positions such as half-kneeling. Encourage weight-shift over the flat foot. Maintain pressure downward into the foot. ■ Progress to static standing activities, then dynamic standing activities.

Child avoids walking barefoot in the grass or sand, wading in water, or playing in the sand or water at the beach or a park.
 	
Child becomes very nervous, anxious, emotionally upset, or aggressive.
	■ Whenever possible, avoid these situations until the child's nervous system is better equipped to handle them.
	
	■ When this is not possible or the child is ready to expand activities:
	
	  ▣ Before the activity, develop a desensitization routine. Start with sustained deep pressure into the feet. The position described above addressing toe-walking is effective. Progress to firm friction massages or compression into the feet, such as jumping on a trampoline.
	
	  ▣ Progress to desensitization of the hands and fingers described above under "Child uses only fingertips."
	
	  ▣ If the child is on the Wilbarger Deep Pressure and Proprioceptive Technique (DPPT) program, initiate treatment before performing the activity.
	
	  ▣ Introduce aversive activities (walking in sand) in a fast but graded progression.
	
	  ▣ Teach the child that these procedures will help him or her overcome the discomfort experienced. Help the child relax. Provide emotional support.

Child has trouble falling asleep.	■ Develop a calming routine prior to bedtime. Include quiet activities or inhibition techniques, such as resistive or deep proprioceptive activities, isometric exercises, modified push-ups, yoga, or other calming activities. ■ Use a heavy comforter, flannel sheets, or a sleeping bag to provide deep-touch input and deep calming.

Gravitational Insecurity: Common Problems and Intervention Strategies

Gravitational insecurity is overresponsiveness to the vestibular system. Anxiety and distress stimulated by movement of the feet off a stable surface or changes in head position that normally would be viewed as nonthreatening. The child has the motor control and balance reactions needed to perform the task, but has an aversive or atypical emotional response.

Child fears walking on uneven surfaces (curbs, gravel, mud, grass).	▪ Provide deep-touch input prior to the activity. ▪ Weight the child's waist to provide deep proprioceptive input and help the child feel more secure. ▪ Provide emotional and physical support.
Child will not sleep in a bed but sleeps on the floor.	▪ Give the child a sleeping bag and a safe corner on the floor to sleep. ▪ Use a weighted blanket.
Child is fearful of heights.	▪ Avoid these positions. The child is not getting accurate information from his or her vestibular-proprioceptive system and is relying on vision. If heights are unavoidable, give deep proprioceptive input (provide steady gentle pressure downward on shoulders) before the activity.
Child screams when lifted or placed on changing table.	▪ Child is fearful of movements into space or backwards. Hold the child firmly and close to your body while moving with him or her, supporting the head and providing deep-touch input.
Child gets carsick.	▪ Seat the child near a window. ▪ Open a window or turn air-conditioner on. Turn vents toward the child. ▪ Give gentle, steady, compressions downward through the head (maintaining alignment), or teach the child to give himself or herself head compressions. ▪ Give the child chewy foods or gum. Try ginger. ▪ Use acupressure wristbands to decrease motion sickness.

Auditory Defensiveness: Common Problems and Intervention Strategies

Auditory defensiveness is the overresponsiveness to normal sound or the registration of auditory input that normally would be ignored or habituated to.

Child covers ears to noises, demonstrates increased anxiety or increased distractibility.	■ Limit extraneous auditory stimuli in the environment. ■ Use rugs or carpet in the area to minimize extraneous auditory stimuli (see chapter 7, Environmental Intervention Techniques). ■ Position the child toward the front of the class to facilitate the child's ability to attend to auditory instructions and block out irrelevant information. ■ Use therapeutic listening techniques (listening to spectrally modulated music through a headset) to decrease hypersensitivity and help to modulate child's nervous system.
Child becomes upset with fire bells or alarms.	■ Forewarn the child of any loud noises before they occur.
Child becomes upset with the noise of a vacuum cleaner.	■ Vacuum when the child is not around. ■ Use a broom, hand sweeper, or electric broom. ■ Prepare the child for the sudden noise. ■ Do not approach child with vacuum cleaner running.
Child becomes upset or agitated in noisy open field or public environments.	■ Avoid special events whenever possible until child's sensory system can accommodate them. ■ Have the child engage in resistive or deep proprioceptive activities before the event to lower resting threshold and increase tolerance. ■ Have the child wear snug clothing or a neoprene vest. ■ Have the child wear earplugs. ■ Use an audiotape player with headphones. Listening to a favorite radio station or CD often will drown out environmental noises and help the child stay focused on an activity. ■ Use therapeutic listening techniques.

Appendix C

Stereotypic and Disruptive Behaviors

Stereotypic, disruptive, and destructive behaviors are often initially provoked by specific events, then they are reinforced and maintained by:

- The sensory stimulation the child receives
- The success encountered within the environment:
  - Effectiveness in meeting the childís needs (calming, arousal, organizing)
  - The attention received (obtained)
  - Termination or acquisition of the activity or event (avoidance)

Behavior	Sensory Input Provided
Rocking	Linear vestibular, rhythmical motion
Spinning self	Rotary vestibular, visual (if eyes are open)
Pacing	Linear vestibular, rhythmic motion, proprioceptive input
Running	Fast vestibular (linear, rotary, or angular depending on direction), proprioceptive
Jumping	Linear vestibular and deep-proprioceptive
Throwing self to floor, crashing, or playing too hard	Vestibular, deep-touch, proprioceptive
Lunging	Vestibular (angular), proprioceptive (especially when stopped by someone)
Head banging	Linear vestibular, vibration, proprioceptive, deep touch, rhythmic motion
Masturbating	Deep-touch pressure, proprioceptive
Hanging upside-down or lying with head inverted	Intense vestibular input
Shaking extremities or hands	Vibration, proprioceptive
Rubbing hands or fisting them together	Deep touch, proprioceptive, visual (if within sight or near face)
End-range fixing or patterning (example: bending wrist, fingers, or elbows into extreme flexion or extension, also seen as knee hyperextension and toe-walking)	Proprioceptive and deep-touch input
Hitting self or others	Deep touch and deep proprioceptive input
Scratching or rubbing	Deep touch and proprioceptive input
Pinching, pushing, or attempting to be pulled	Deep touch and proprioceptive input
Finger flicking	Visual, some proprioceptive input

(*continued*)

205

Stereotypic and Disruptive Behaviors (*Continued*)

Behavior	Sensory Input Provided
Eyes: end-range fixing or angling, crossing eyes, or overconvergence of eyes	Proprioceptive from end-range fixing, visual
Spinning objects	Rotary vestibular and visual (visual-vestibular integration)
Mouthing clothes and objects	Proprioceptive and tactile. Gustatory if the objects have a flavor
Chewing on clothes or items	Deep proprioceptive and deep touch
Teeth grinding	Deep proprioceptive, vestibular from the vibration, auditory
Biting self or others	Deep proprioceptive, deep-touch input
Presses hand to mouth or teeth firmly	Deep proprioceptive and deep-touch input
Ear flicking	Vestibular (vibration and sound), proprioceptive, and tactile
Covers ears	Auditory
Humming, singing, self-talk, and other quiet, steady vocalizations	Rhythmic auditory and vibration, proprioceptive from generating vocalization the vocalizations
Screaming nonstop	Auditory and vestibular
Smelling and sniffing objects	Olfactory and gustatory; strong systemic input

Appendix D

Analyzing Behavior Worksheet

Child's name _____

Date _____

Behavior _____

Define the behavior:

Are Behaviors Linked? (Yes/No)

☐ Y ☐ N Stem from the same cause?

☐ Y ☐ N Occur in a predictable pattern?

Group behaviors with the same cause together.

Analyze behaviors with the same underlying cause as one behavior (a single entity).

Priority for change:

☐ Harmful to self or others

☐ Destructive

☐ Disruptive/Interferes with learning

☐ Not acceptable (socially)

Antecedent: Is it a problem? (Yes/No)

☐ Y ☐ N Size of room

☐ Y ☐ N Structured/unstructured task

☐ Y ☐ N Adult-child ratio?

☐ Y ☐ N Environmental factors: Noise/clutter/other

☐ Y ☐ N Time of day:

☐ Y ☐ N Morning/evening/transitions?

☐ Y ☐ N During certain activities?

Characteristics of activity:

What activity or event preceded the behavior?

Recent special events

☐ Illness

☐ Lack of sleep

☐ Family dispute

☐ Other:

☐ None

Warning signs

☐ Restlessness

☐ Eye aversion

☐ Distractibility

☐ Pause

☐ Raises voice

☐ Self-stimulation or repetitive pattern: Describe behavior

☐ Other:

Action Plan

☐ Stop

☐ Alter

☐ Limit or modify the behavior

☐ Ignore

☐ Treat the underlying problem

Action Plan

Environmental changes needed:

Action Plan

Is a referral to a professional indicated?

Action Plan

Can you intervene at this point to ward off the behavior?

Child's name _____

Date _____

Analyzing Behavior Worksheet (continued)

Behavior _____

Define the behavior:

Primary cause: Obtain

☐ Attention
☐ Object
☐ Need
☐ Want
☐ Activity
☐ Sensory
  ☐ productive
  ☐ nonproductive

Does it work for the child?

Is the child successful in obtaining what he wants/needs?

Action Plan

Identify a method to get what the child wants as part of his normal schedule, as a reward, etc.

Primary Cause: Avoid

☐ Attention
  ☐ positive
  ☐ negative
☐ People
☐ Situations
☐ Transitions
☐ Task, object or activity

Action Plan

Perform task analysis

☐ Task too difficult?
☐ Task not stimulating?
☐ Not challenging?
☐ Task boring?
☐ Difficulty adjusting to transition?
☐ Task overwhelming?
☐ Dislikes task?
☐ Lacks self-confidence?
☐ Fears task?
☐ Avoids sensory aspect?
☐ Task has no meaning?

Perform skills analysis

Does child have the necessary skills to do the task?

If not, how will you remediate?

Analyze emotional response

If child has necessary skills, give emotional support and physical assistance.

Primary Cause: Avoiding Sensory
(Internal Systemic)

What type of sensory input?

☐ Vestibular
☐ Auditory
☐ Visual
☐ Smell
☐ Tactile

Is it systemic/visceral due to:

☐ Pain or discomfort?
☐ Hunger?
☐ Illness or impending illness?
☐ Hot, tired, sweaty?
☐ Other: _____

Is he avoiding something sensory from the environment? Identify the cause:

Action Plan

1. Identify if sensory and how you will remediate.

2. If based upon a need, can you rectify it?

Social and Communication—Aspects of Behavior

☐ Y ☐ N **Is it socially acceptable?**

If not, identify other methods.

☐ Y ☐ N **Is method of communication acceptable?**

If not, must address communication strategies.

Primary Causes: Action Plan

☐ Socially Acceptable Behaviors: Teach
☐ Communication Strategies: Identify and teach
☐ Task: Alter, modify, or assist
☐ Skills: Teach or develop skills
☐ Sensory Options:
☐ Enhance the sensory component
☐ Decrease sensory component
☐ Provide sensory diets
☐ Provide scheduled sensory activities
☐ Environmental Modifications:

Analyzing Behavior Worksheet (continued)

Define the behavior:

Consequence to Behavior:

What predicts the behavior?

What promotes the behavior?

What happened after the behavior?

What are consequences to behavior?

What is primary cause?

What is primary reinforcer?

What are secondary reinforcers?

Action Plan

What behavior do you want to occur?

Stop/Alter/Limit/Modify the Behavior/Do nothing or treat the underlying cause.

Environmental changes needed?

What communication strategies are needed?

What modifications to task and skills will you make?

When will you intervene?

Is a sensory diet needed?

What reinforcers will you use?

What consequences will there be?

What behavioral strategies will you use?

Do you need to refer the child for other services?
OT or PT for sensory integration therapy or other services?

Appendix E

Intervention for Challenging Behaviors

```
                                                    ┌──────────────┐
                                                    │    Obtain    │
                                                    └──────────────┘
```

Social/Communication

Attention
- Smiles, hugs, praise
- Negative attention
- Shock/surprise reaction
- Full ownership

Intervention

Give structured, positive attention to desired on-task behaviors

Negative attention-seeking behaviors:
- Behavioral intervention techniques
- Ignore negative behaviors
- Control the responses of others in the area
- Intervene before negative behavior begins; praise on-task behavior
- Educate all team members
- Be consistent, implement in all environments

Full Ownership Behaviors

Constructive
- Serves a goal or purpose
- Increased compliance, participation or motivation is seen
- No intervention

Destructive
- Teach situations not allowed
- Be consistent in enforcing
- Reinforce desired behavior
- Reinforce before undesirable behaviors are displayed
- Use delayed-gratification techniques
- Keep child engaged in task

Need or want—object or activity
- Personal need (food, drink, toilet)
- Preferred object or activity
- Need or want

Intervention

Identify what is being communicated
Is the method of communicating acceptable?

If Acceptable
No intervention

If Unacceptable
Is the child able to know what he or she needs or wants?

If Yes
- Establish communication
- Implement communication system
- Be consistent
- Implement in all environments
- Teach child acceptable methods of communicating
- Teach delayed gratification for need or want

If No
- Anticipate needs
- Control environment
- Teach coping skills

O

Obtain

Internalized/Systemic

Sensory Input

Productive
- Underresponsive system
- Stimulate sensory processing, registration, or organization
- Increase arousal, pleasure, or postural tone

Nonproductive
- Endorphin release
- Self stimulation without a purpose

Intervention

Intervention

If Acceptable
No intervention

If Unacceptable
Intervention

- Analyze to determine sensory need being met
- Identify acceptable alternative activities that meet the sensory need
- Design a sensory-based program and regimen
- Modify activities for enhanced sensory feedback
- Teach and prompt the child to use the alternative activities
- Be consistent; implement in all environments
- Use behavior modification techniques to extinguish, alter, or limit unacceptable behaviors

Intervention for Challenging Behaviors

```
                                                    ┌─────────────────┐
                                                    │  Avoid/Escape   │
                                                    └─────────────────┘
                        ┌──────────────────────┐
                        │    Communication     │
                        └──────────────────────┘
```

Attention
- New people – new situations
- Negative attention
- Reprimands

Intervention
Give structured positive attention to desired on-task behaviors

Teach
- Routine greetings
- Social skills
- Pragmatics and appropriate social and interaction skills

Prepare the child for the new situations
- Teach skills needed
- Familiarize the child with all aspects of new situation
- Practice related activities and responses
- Prompt desired behaviors and actions
- Reinforce desired behavior

Task, object, activity
Child avoids object, activity

Intervention
Identify aspect of task child is trying to avoid

Task Analysis	Skills Analysis	Emotional Analysis
Determine skills needed to accomplish task	Assess child's skills	Analyze child's emotional response

Task Too Difficult
- Modifiy task to make it easier. Provide emotional support
- Do not change activity; provide assistance and emotional support
- Provide therapeutic intervention to improve skills

Task boring, not stimulating or challenging
- Modify task to make it more difficult or demanding
- Enhance sensory feedback in task or instructions
- Increase stimulation to activity

Task has no meaning
- Increase sensory registration
- Attach meaning to the activity
- Connect the idea of the task to its end product
- Increase sensory feedback

Task overwhelming
- Modify task and environment to decrease stimulation
- Break task into manageable pieces; increase organization of task

Dislikes task
- Prompt: Praise and reward task completion

Avoids task due to sensory component
- Treat underlying sensory defensiveness using SI principles
- Refer to sensory avoiding

Difficulty adjusting to transition
- Establish systems and routines
- Refer to (chapter 5) Systems to increase performance

Lacks self-confidence
- Provide emotional support during task completion

Fear of task
- If rational: Refer to "Task too Difficult." Otherwise, refer to "Avoid: Internal Systemic Sensory."

A

Avoid/Escape

Internalized/Systemic

Sensory
- Overarousal
- Overstimulated
- Modulation disorders
  - Auditory • Visual • Tactile • Postural
  - Olfactory (Smell)
  - Attempts to calm and organize

Systemic/Visceral
- Pain or discomfort
- Hunger
- Autoimmune response and histamine reactions
- Illness or impending illness
- Hot, tired, or sweaty

Intervention

Intervention

Identify sensory systems and aspect of the environment contributing to overload
- Decrease environmental stimulation

Assist parents to differentiate between sensory-based versus medically-based concerns

Identify appropriate and effective, calming and organizing, sensory-based activities
- Teach child to identify warning signs of escalating stress and overload
- Teach child to recognize and communicate feelings
- Teach alternate activity for calming
- Guide child to use alternate activities
- Integrate calming sensory-based activities into child's schedule

Teach child to recognize signs of internal body reactions

Remediate underlying modulation difficulty

Refer to appropriate medical professional

Systematically increase tolerance for and scope of new activities

References

Ayres, J. A. 1972. *Sensory integration and learning disorders.* Los Angeles: Western Psychological Services.

Ayres, J. A. 1979. *Sensory integration and the child.* Los Angeles: Western Psychological Services.

Bundy, A., S. Lane, and E. Murray. 2002. *Sensory integration theory and practice.* 2nd ed. Philadelphia: F. A. Davis Company.

Charlop, M. H., and I. K. Haymes. 1996. Using obsessions as reinforcers with and without mild reductive procedures to decrease autistic children's inappropriate behaviors. *Journal of Autism and Developmental Disorders* 26:527–46.

Charlop, M. H., P. F. Kurtz, and F. Casey. 1990. Using aberrant behavior as reinforcers for autistic children. *Journal of Applied Behavioral Analysis* 23:163–81.

Cipani, E. 1998. Three behavioral functions of classroom noncompliance: Diagnostic and treatment implications. *Focus on Autism and Other Developmental Disabilities* 13 (2): 66–72.

Coffey, D. S. 1998. Self-organization, complexity and chaos: The new biology for medicine. *Nature Medicine* 4 (8): 882–85.

Dunn, W. 1999. *Sensory Profile.* San Antonio, TX: The Psychological Corporation.

Durand, V. M. 1990. Severe behavioral problems: A functional communication training approach. New York: Teachers College Press.

Epstein, L., M. T. Taubman, and O. I. Lovaas. 1985. Changes in self-stimulatory behavior with treatment. *Journal of Abnormal Child Psychology* 13:281–94.

Favell, J. E., and J. W. Greene. 1981. *How to treat self-injurious behavior.* Austin, TX: Pro-Ed.

Florida Department of Education. 2001. Technical Assistant Paper (10967). *Auditory Processing Disorders.* Paper Number FY 2001-9. Division of Public Schools and Community Education 850:488–1106.

Gray, C. 1994. *The original social storybook,* Arlington, TX: Future Horizons, http://www.thegraycenter.org.

Gray, J. A. 1982. *The neurophysiology of anxiety.* Oxford: Clarendon Press.

Gubbay, S. S. 1975. *The clumsy child.* Philadelphia: W. B. Saunders.

Haron, M. 1999. Understanding sensory integrative dysfunction. *Twins Magazine,* Nov./Dec.

Katz, J., and L. Wilde. 1994. Auditory processing disorders. In *Handbook of clinical audiology.* 4th ed. edited by J. Katz, 409. Baltimore: Williams & Wilkins.

Kimball, J. G. 1999. Sensory integration frame of reference. In *Frames of reference for pediatric occupation therapy.* 2nd ed. edited by P. Kramer and J. Hinojosa. Baltimore: Lippincott Williams & Wilkins.

Koomar J., and A. Bundy. 2002. Creating direct intervention from theory. In *Sensory integration and practice.* 2nd ed. edited by A. Bundy, S. Lane, and E. Murray, 261–306. Philadelphia: F. A. Davis.

LaGrossa, J. 2003. Uncovering OCD: Does it have connection to sensory integrative disorder? *Advance for Physical Therapists & Assistants,* Aug. 4.

Lovaas, O. I., I. Schreibman, R., Koegel, and R. Rehm. 1971. Selective responding by autistic children to multiple sensory input. *Journal of Abnormal Psychology* 77 (3): 211–22.

Lovaas, O., C. Newsom, and C. Hickman. 1987. Self-stimulatory behavior and perception of reinforcement. *Journal of Applied Behavioral Analysis* 20:45–68.

Luce, S. C., and W. P. Christian. 1981 *How to reduce autistic and severely maladaptive behaviors.* Austin, TX: Pro-Ed.

Mace, F. C., M. L. Hock, J. S. Lalli, B. J. West, P. Belfiore, E. Pinter, and D. K. Brown. 1988. Behavioral momentum in the treatment of non-compliance. *Journal of Applied Behavior Analysis* 21:123–41.

Maurice, C., G. Green, and S. C. Luce. 1996. *Behavioral intervention for young children with autism.* Austin, TX: Pro-Ed.

Mercer, C. D., and M. E. Snell. 1977. Learning theory in mental retardation: Implication for teaching. Columbus, OH: Merrill.

Miller, L. J., J. Wilbarger, T. Stackhouse, and S. Trunnell. 2002. Use of clinical reasoning in occupational therapy: The STEP-SI model of intervention of sensory modulation dysfunction. In *Sensory integration and practice.* 2nd ed. edited by A. Bundy, S. Lane and E. Murray, 435–51. Philadelphia: F. A. Davis.

Mulligan, S. 2003. Examination of the evidence for occupational therapy using a sensory integrative framework for children: Part one. *Sensory Integration* 26 (1).

Murray-Slutsky, C., and B. Paris. 2000. *Exploring the spectrum of autism and pervasive developmental disorders.* San Antonio, TX: Therapy Skill Builders.

O'Neil, R. E., R. H. Horner, R. Albin, K. Storey, and J. Sprague. 1990. *Functional assessment of problem behavior: A practical guide.* Pacific Grove, CA: Brooks/Cole.

Oetter, P., E. W. Richter, and S. M. Frick. 1995. M.O.R.E.: *Integrating the mouth with sensory and postural functions.* Hugo, MN: PDP Press.

Parham, L. D., and Z. Mailloux. 2001. Sensory integration, In *Occupational therapy for children.* 4th ed. edited by J. Case-Smith, A. S. Allen, and P. N. Pratt, St Louis: Mosby.

Roley, S. S., E. I. Blanche, and R. C. Shaaf. 2001. *Understanding the nature of sensory integration with diverse populations.* San Antonio, TX: Therapy Skill Builders.

Royeen, C. B. 2003. The 2003 Eleanor Clarke Slagle Lecture. Chaotic occupational therapy: Collective wisdom for a complex profession. *The American Journal of Occupational Therapy* 57 (6): 609–24.

Trott, M. C., M. Laurel, and S. Windeck, S. 1993. *SenseAbilities: Understanding sensory integration.* San Antonio, TX: Therapy Skill Builders.

Vygotsky, L. S. 1978. *Mind in society.* Cambridge, MA: Harvard University Press.

Wilbarger, P. 1984. Planning an adequate sensory diet: Application of sensory processing theory during the first year of life. *Zero to Three* 5 (1): 7–12.

———. 1995. The sensory diet: Activity programs based on sensory processing theory. *Sensory Integration Special Interest Section Newsletter* 18 (2):1–4.

Wilbarger, P., and J. Wilbarger. 1991. *Sensory defensiveness in children aged 2–12.* Santa Barbara, CA: Avanti Educational Programs.

Williams, M. S., and S. Shellenberger. 1996. How does your engine run? A leader's guide to the Alert program for self-regulation. Albuquerque, NM: TherapyWorks.

———. 2001. *Take five! Staying alert at home and school.* Albuquerque, NM: TherapyWorks.

Additional readings

Ayres, J. A. 1972. Improving academic scores through sensory integration. *Journal of Learning Disabilities* 5:338–43.

Barlow, J, and S. Stewart-Brown. 2000. Behavior problems and group-based parent education programs. *Developmental and Behavioral Pediatrics* 21 (5): 356–70.

Graffam, B. 2003. Constructivism and Understanding: Implementing the Teaching for Understanding Framework. *The Journal of Secondary Gifted Education* 15 (1): 13–22.

Hanft, B., L. J. Miller, and S. Lane. 2000. Toward a consensus in terminology in sensory integration theory and practice, Part 3: Observable Behaviors: Sensory Integrative Dysfunction. *Sensory Integration Special Interest Section Quarterly* 23 (3).

Kranowitz, C. 1998. *The Out-of-Sync Child: Recognizing and coping with sensory integrative dysfunction.* New York: Skylight Press.

Parham, D. 1998. The relationship of sensory integrative development to achievement in elementary students: Four year longitudinal patterns. *Occupational Therapy Journal of Research* 18 (3): 105–27.

Pfeiffer, B. 2002. The impact of sensory integration on occupations in childhood through adulthood: A case study. *Sensory Integration Special Interest Section Quarterly* 25 (1).

Zuckerman B. S., et al. 1999. Infancy and toddler years. In *Developmental-Behavioral Pediatrics.* 3rd ed. edited by M. D. Levine et al. Philadelphia: W. B. Saunders.